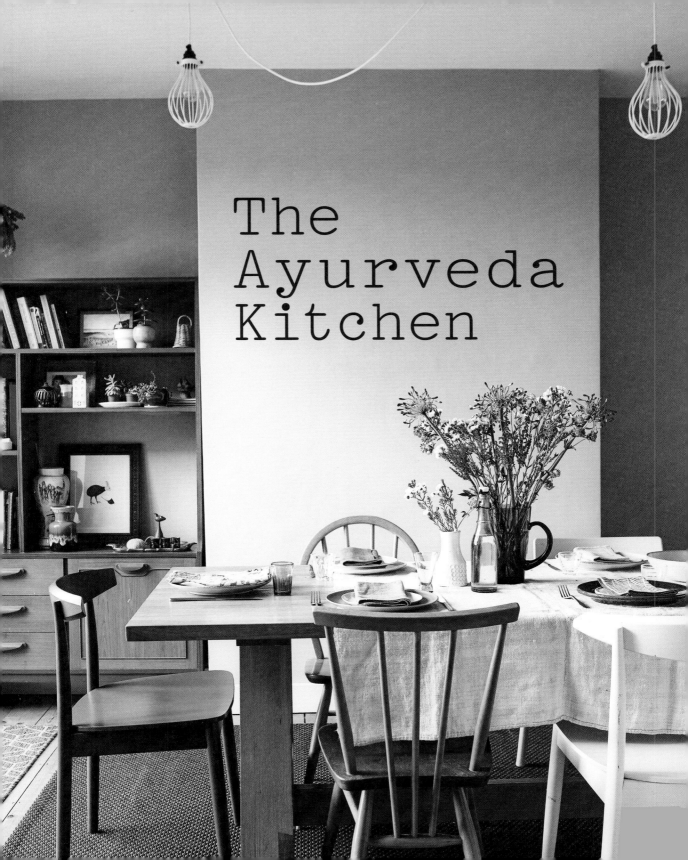

The Ayurveda Kitchen

To Will and our two girls, who encouraged, shaped and blew life into this book.

First published in Great Britain in 2021 by Aster, an imprint of Octopus Publishing Group Ltd, Carmelite House, 50 Victoria Embankment, London EC4Y 0DZ
www.octopusbooks.co.uk
www.octopusbooksusa.com

An Hachette UK Company
www.hachette.co.uk

Text copyright © Anne Heigham 2021
Design & layout copyright © Octopus Publishing Group Ltd 2021
Photography copyright © Yuki Suguira 2021

Distributed in the US by Hachette Book Group, 1290 Avenue of the Americas, 4th and 5th Floors, New York, NY 10104

Distributed in Canada by Canadian Manda Group, 664 Annette St, Toronto, Ontario, Canada M6S 2C8

ISBN 978-1-78325-361-6

A CIP catalogue record for this book is available from the British Library.

Printed and bound in China.

10 9 8 7 6 5 4 3 2 1

Publisher's note

All reasonable care has been taken in the preparation of this book but the information it contains is not intended to take the place of treatment by a qualified medical practitioner.

Before making any changes in your health regime, always consult a doctor. You must seek professional advice if you are in any doubt about any medical condition. Any application of the ideas and information contained in this book is at the reader's sole discretion and risk.

Neither Octopus Publishing Group Limited or the author take any responsibility for any consequences resulting from the use or misuse of information contained in this book.

Cook's notes

Standard level spoon measurements are used in all recipes. 1 tablespoon = one 15ml spoon. 1 teaspoon = one 5ml spoon

Eggs should be medium unless otherwise stated.

Milk should be full fat unless otherwise stated.

Ovens should be preheated to the specific temperature given.

Consultant Publisher: Kate Adams
Art Director: Yasia Williams-Leedham
Senior Editor: Leanne Bryan
Copy Editor: Salima Hirani
Designer: Leonardo Collina
Photographer: Yuki Suguira
Props Stylist: Alexander Breeze
Food Stylist: Marina Filippelli
Illustrator: Abi Read
Assistant Production Manager: Lucy Carter

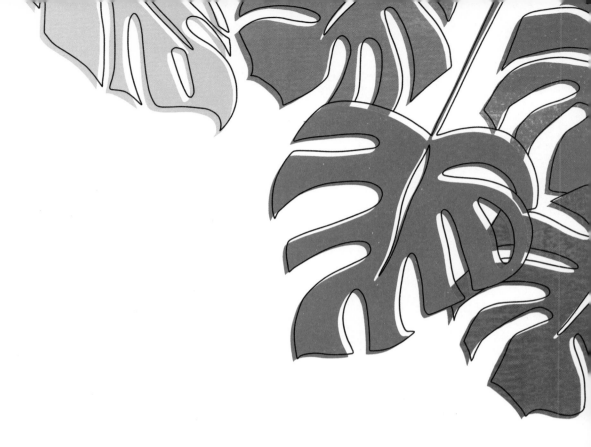

The Ayurveda Kitchen

Transform your kitchen into a sanctuary for health –
with 80 perfectly balanced recipes

Anne Heigham

Contents

Foreword

There are few things as enjoyable as eating a delicious meal, and when you know the food on your plate is bringing you closer to a state of harmony and balance, it is even more pleasurable.

I am a complementary health practitioner and I love to cook. In my Ayurvedic clinic I see people from all walks of life who are suffering from chronic complaints, such as asthma, digestive problems, lethargy and general poor health. They usually come to me because they have heard I have an unusual way of helping people to feel better. In essence, my approach is simple – it involves eating and it involves breathing. And it is underpinned by the principles of Ayurveda.

Developed more than 5,000 years ago in India, Ayurveda is one of the world's oldest healing systems. This Sanskrit word translates as 'science of life'. The discipline has evolved over the millennia, so while its principles are ancient, the practice still has much to offer us in the 21st century. Indeed, recent scientific advances are proving the efficacy of these age-old approaches.

I spent many years training to be an Ayurvedic practitioner in the UK and India, and am one of a very small number of advanced specialist practitioners in the UK. There are multiple sources of information out there if you want to delve into the details of Ayurveda. I find too much information can sometimes get in the way of moving forwards in life so, on pages 12–21, I explain enough of the basic principles to give you a working understanding of the discipline. At its core is the belief that health and wellness depend on a delicate balance between the mind, body

and spirit. The main goal of the practice is to promote good health and prevent illnesses from taking hold. Our bodies are complex mechanisms that rely on each part working well – if you are out of kilter in one area, this will impact another. Guided by Ayurvedic principles, you can achieve and maintain internal balance, enabling you to live your life in a state of harmony.

In this book I aim to help you use Ayurvedic culinary practices in your everyday life in the space that is at the heart of your home – the kitchen. In these pages I share with you much of the wisdom I have absorbed over the years through my clinical practice, to guide you in transforming your kitchen into a wellness space that will lift your spirit, improve your health and help you to bring more balance to your life. If you follow the concepts in this book you should be able to enhance your overall health and wellbeing within four to six weeks.

As both an Ayurvedic practitioner and yoga teacher, I have spent many years treating clients with dietary and supplement advice, therapeutic massage treatments and techniques to enhance mental clarity. This holistic approach requires the client to do the work, with my assistance, to bring about a change in their life, which is empowering for them. The great thing about this approach is that, once people start making changes that help them to feel better, they generally tend to stick with them. It becomes a way of life

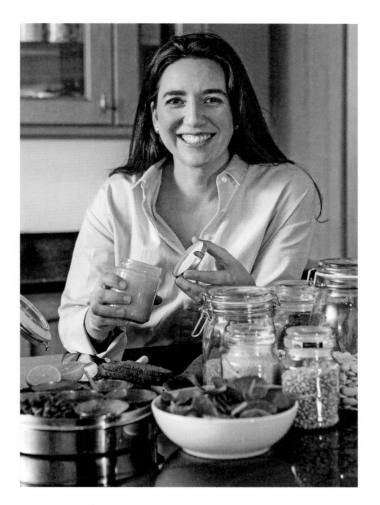

and, because they feel better, there is rarely the desire to go back to eating and living in other ways – it just does not appeal to them anymore. And if they do go off track for a while (which is not a problem), they tend to notice the difference in how they feel, which propels them to return to what makes them feel better.

Over the years I have been repeatedly asked to provide recipes to support the advice I give in my clinics. I love to cook and, over time, have created many recipes in which I apply the core principles of Ayurveda. I have seen so often the positive effect that eating this way can have on our overall state of health, and from this, *The Ayurveda Kitchen* was born. I hope this book inspires you to get creative in your kitchen and I wish you much enjoyment on your culinary journey.

Anne Heigham

What is the Ayurveda Kitchen?

The concept of the Ayurveda Kitchen is born out of the Ayurvedic tradition, in which the kitchen is considered a sacred space, a source of deep nourishment and healing. Given the right guidance and attention, you can transform your own kitchen into a harmonious wellness sanctuary in which you can create delicious and health-giving meals.

The Ayurveda Kitchen is a vibrant space that you feel motivated to be in and can ultimately thrive in. A person's equilibrium is affected by many factors, both internal and external. Consequently, there are many facets to the Ayurveda Kitchen, which fall within three main considerations – the environment itself, the ingredients you use in it and the way in which you use the space.

The environment

The Ayurveda Kitchen engages all the senses. Imagine fresh, vibrant herbs growing, seeds sprouting and pickles fermenting, clean organized cupboards with delicious aromatic spice mixes, and clear worktops ready for preparing super-fresh vegetables. Less is more in this space – one good knife, sharpened with care, a big beautiful chopping board and a few good pots and pans are all you need. By lovingly caring for our kitchen space, we can make cooking within it easier and more enticing. Just as we would not want to leave waste in a sacred space, we want our kitchen to be uplifting, free of clutter and debris, a space of clear, clean energy. On pages 22–25 I show you how to turn any available space into an Ayurveda Kitchen and maintain it in a way that nurtures the space that nurtures you.

The ingredients

In the Ayurveda Kitchen, there is reduced waste, chemicals and packaged foods, which is good for you and the environment. It becomes a space for the seasons, for nature – after all, it is nature that provides our food. Seasonal eating underpins the Ayurveda Kitchen, and keeps us close to the natural rhythms that we are connected to, helping to maintain internal balance as well as balance within the external world. On pages 48–65, I outline the Ayurvedic approach to seasonal cooking and provide practical guidelines on using your Ayurveda Kitchen within the different seasons.

Using the space

In the Ayurvedic tradition, the consciousness of the chef is one of the main ingredients in any meal. The kitchen is a creative space in which we can transform loving thoughts into nourishment, and it is believed that the energy this imparts to the food contributes to its healing properties. On pages 34–38, I suggest ways in which you can bring more consciousness into your kitchen. Equally, bringing mindfulness to the way in which you eat your meals (see pages 39–43) improves digestion.

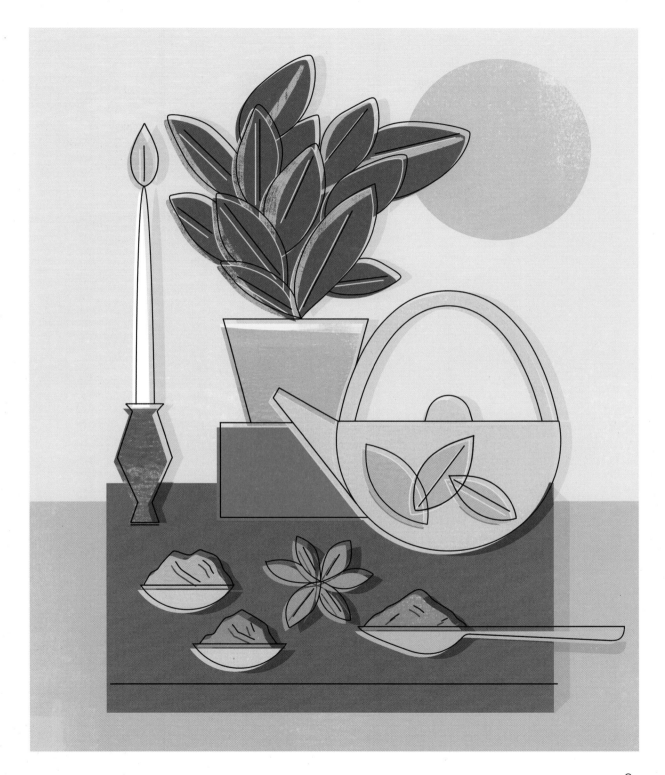

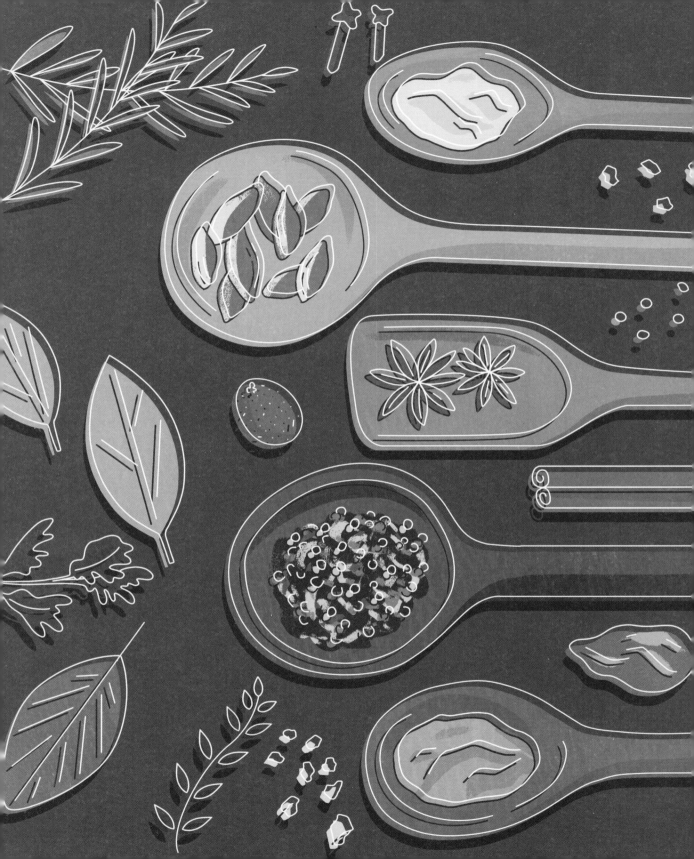

As you are in your kitchen regularly, it is a great space in which to be more conscious about your breath, posture and movement, all of which serve to improve your metabolism and the quality of your life force. I have seen the power of effective breathing patterns on physical, mental and emotional fitness, so my approach incorporates the art of breathing and how to experience this in your kitchen (see pages 44–5). We can then use the kitchen as a trigger to remember how to breathe and be.

The recipes

Once you have set up your Ayurveda Kitchen, you can begin creating nourishing, delicious and balancing meals for you and your loved ones. I have included in this book 80 recipes that are naturally balanced, from an Ayurvedic viewpoint, along with a few ideas for spinning many of these off in different directions, depending on the seasons and your taste preferences. Once the basic principles become familiar, over time you will find you are able to create your own Ayurveda-inspired recipes. Using the guiding principles of when, how and what to eat, the potential for wellness is brought to life through your hands in your kitchen.

Each of the recipes has been designed to help create balance in the body and provide nutrients we all need for healthy tissue. Ayurveda takes account of the way certain spices react with certain ingredients so that each works optimally. In the recipes I aim for a greater bio-availability of the important constituents, to give you the best chance of assimilating those nutrients effectively. But it is important to bear in mind that we are complex individuals and do not always fit into convenient categories. Your digestive system is unique and the reason you prefer certain foods is also unique. This is often related to your life-long experiences with food and emotions as well as your own instinctive taste preferences.

Ayurveda is an excellent base from which to observe the effects of particular foods on you, both positive and negative, so I actively encourage you to play with the recipes and switch-up ingredients to those you favour and know work well with you and your body. However, it is also important to remain open minded towards the effect certain foods have on you. As the digestive fire (see page 18) improves, we often find we are able to tolerate foods that we could not previously.

'Let food be your first medicine and the kitchen your first pharmacy.'

Taittiriya Upanishad

11

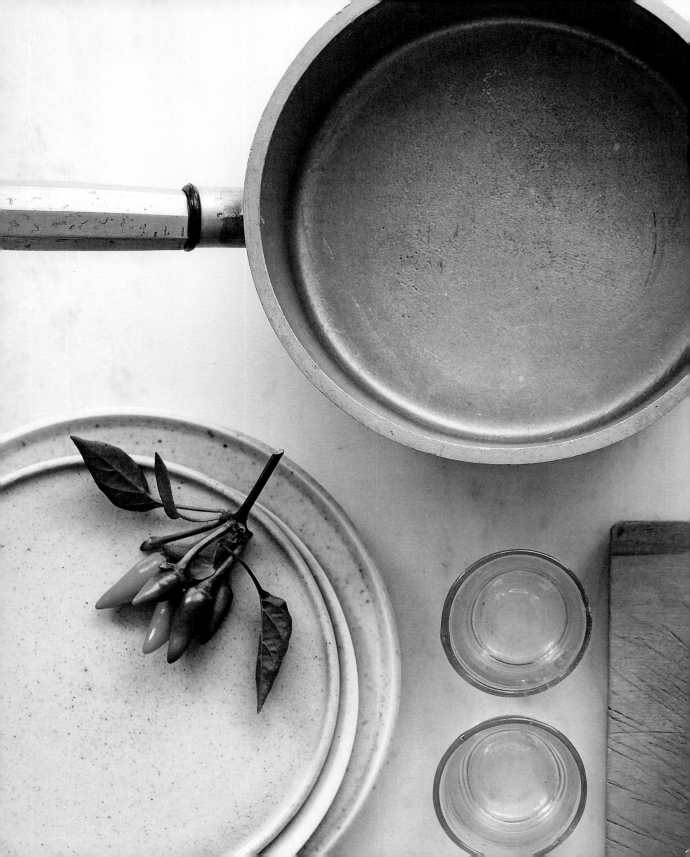

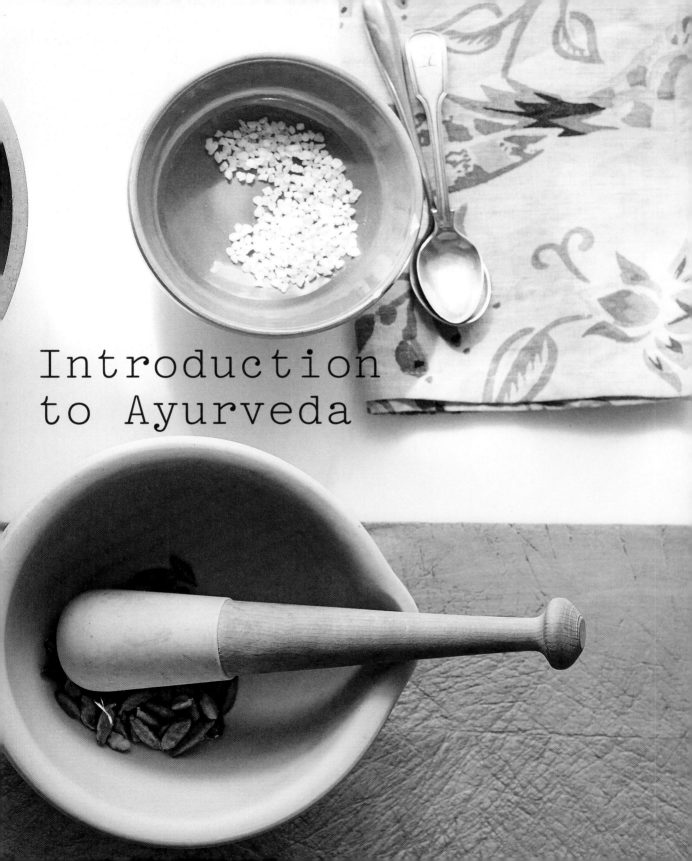

Introduction
to Ayurveda

Science of life _____

At its heart, Ayurveda is a truly holistic science – it works on the principle that what we think, what we feel and how we live all have an impact on our health and longevity.

Building blocks of matter

According to Ayurveda, there are three dynamic energies that give rise to all physical matter, each with a different nature. These three energies influence the mode of action of all matter, and each is a necessary part of life. These energies are represented in us, particularly in the action of the mind, but also in the body.

Sattva **(harmony)** This is the energy of a beautiful piece of classical music or mantra. When you experience this energy, lots of oxytocin and dopamine freely circulate. It is a state of equanimity, following the natural rhythm and harmony of everything, and is driven by love and kindness.

Rajas **(drive)** *Rajas* is the energy of pumped-up rock music. It is often fuelled by adrenaline and cortisol, and there is more lust, anger, desire, greed and energy pumping through the veins.

Tamas **(inertia)** This is the energy of a laid-back, sorrowful acoustic riff. It is lower in dopamine and serotonin, higher in laziness. This energy often expresses itself as a mañana/procrastinating approach to life, unhappiness and sleepiness.

These three energies combine in varying levels within all aspects of the material world. The material world is built from five elements: earth (from *tamas*), water, fire (from *rajas*), air and ether (space from *sattva*). Each of these elements or states has its own type of energy, which defines the nature of the matter made from it. This is a core principle in Ayurveda and is applied to understanding everything – people, diseases, food, seasons, the environment, activities, and so on.

Doshas are conceptual models representing three different blends of the elements, giving each *dosha* a specific set of qualities or *gunas* (see below).

Kapha
Combination of Water and earth.

Characteristics Cold, heavy, moist, soft, stable, slimy.

Pitta
Combination of Fire and water.

Characteristics Hot, light, sharp, moist, liquid, mobile.

Vata
Combination of Air and ether.

Characteristics Cold, dry, light, rough, mobile, subtle, non-slimy.

The 20 *gunas*

In Ayurveda these opposing qualities (see box, opposite) are applied to maintain balance within the triad of life (mind, body and soul). In general terms, this means that if a thing is too hot, you apply something cooling to counter the excessive heating effect (this usually takes place through mechanisms such as alkalizing the pH or introducing an anti-inflammatory property). If something has become very dry, you add something moistening to alleviate the dryness. So in cooking, if you are making a cake or some dough and the mixture is looking too dry, you would add more liquid to obtain an ideal consistency. These principles can be applied in the rest of life as readily as they can in the kitchen to reach an optimum point of balance.

The *gunas*

All matter has one or a combination of these qualities, which exist in ten pairs of opposites.

- Hot – Cold
- Heavy – Light
- Dull – Sharp
- Moist – Dry
- Smooth – Rough
- Solid – Liquid
- Soft – Hard
- Stable – Mobile
- Gross – Subtle
- Slimy – Non-slimy

Prakruti (individual constitution)

We are all born into the world with our unique set of genes, which gives us our physical and mental constitution and characteristics, or *prakruti*, as it is known in Ayurveda. Each person's *prakruti* will fall under a specific *dosha* or combination of *doshas*. Everyone has all the five elements in them, but some elements are likely to be more dominant than others. You may, for example, have a dominance of fire, water, and earth, which means you will have certain traits that are associated with these elements.

Furthermore, as we move through our lives, we are affected by the interactions we have with our external environment, which is also comprised of the five elements. These interactions cause a move away from your original *prakruti*. Some of this movement has its origins in our life in the womb, while life outside the womb, with its traumatic experiences, injuries, viruses, inappropriate dietary and lifestyle patterns, and so on, will go on to affect each person. These interactions cause different elements to increase, decrease or become disrupted, and this imbalance from our original state can set us on a path to ill-health.

Determining your *prakruti*

To determine your own *prakruti* can be challenging. I would advise anyone to consult a qualified practitioner who can perform a pulse diagnosis (we feel pulses very differently to Western medicine in Ayurveda) to determine your *prakruti* accurately. Over the years there have been countless instances in which I have formed an idea of a client's *prakruti* based on their appearance and what they tell me about themselves, only to find, on taking their pulse, that it is actually completely different.

For example, I have had clients with a very low BMI, erratic concentration and thinking patterns and erratic hunger, all pointing to a *vata*-dominant constitution. However, on taking their pulse I have found they are actually *kapha*-dominant, which is at the other end of the scale. Traumatic experiences or prolonged periods of physical or psychological stress had led to the implementation of particular dietary and lifestyle regimes. Coupled with metabolic changes, these had led to significant weight loss and a different way of being, resulting in an appearance altogether different to how it would be in their normal balanced state. The state of imbalance here is referred to as *vikruti*, which is much easier to identify than *prakruti*.

In the example above, I would aim to address the underlying cause of the psychological stress, improve the digestive functioning and gently nourish the individual in order to soothe the elevated *vata* (air and ether elements), which would naturally lead them back towards the natural state of *kapha* (water and earth elements). To work on the body, mind and spirit, I would do this with a range of techniques, including: food recommendations that are warm in temperature and taste and are grounding and nourishing; lifestyle changes that are likely to encourage the individual to slow down; herb supplements to relieve negative impacts of prolonged stress; warm therapeutic oil treatments; and meditation/yoga instruction.

Rebalancing

In order to rebalance the scales, Ayurveda seeks to use opposing (and, occasionally, similar) qualities to influence imbalances. Foods or herbs that can be ascribed specific *gunas* or qualities (see page 15) that oppose

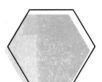
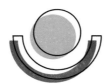
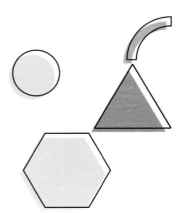

the characteristics of the imbalance are used to remedy the situation.

For example, if your skin is rough and dry, it needs something smooth and moist added to it, such as more oil, both internally and externally. If you always feel cold, you need to eat more food that is warm in both flavour and temperature. If you feel your thoughts are too mobile (that you are always jumping from one thought to the next), following stable patterns, such as sitting down daily to meditate at a regular time, can help to stabilize the thought processes. And if your body feels heavy and dull, you need to eat foods that are lighter in both quality and quantity, and foods with a sharper, pungent taste (see page 48).

This sounds quite simplistic, but when you look into the constituents or properties of many herbs or treatments, often you will find there is modern science that underpins these processes. For example, ginger root is used widely in Ayurveda to promote good *agni* digestion (see page 18) and calm excessive *vata*. It is light, oily, pungent and heating in nature – qualities that come from its constituents, such as gingerols

and shogaols. Ginger's incredible *agni*-boosting ability has been researched in great detail and it has been shown to possess free radical-scavenging, antioxidant and inhibition of lipid peroxidation activities[1], and has been subject to several double-blind placebo trials for the treatment of Type 2 diabetes[2, 3] that have verified its efficacy in improving this condition through how it works on the digestive system as a whole.

Agni (metabolic fire) and *prana* (life force)

When we strip our understanding of a human being back to a simple level, our cells require oxygen, water and nutrients from foods for them to perform their functions, reproduce and sustain life. The conversion of all these building blocks into fuel for our lives happens via our metabolism, known as *agni* (metabolic fire) and our *prana* (life force). Ayurveda enables us to maintain and encourage good metabolism. It works on the principle that we are not just a collection of cells that operates autonomously, but on the premise that there is something that drives this operation. We can call that the soul (*atman*) or the non-material aspect of us. This is a fundamentally

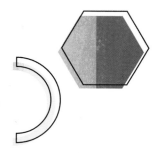

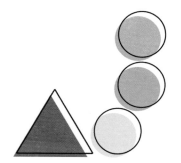

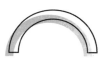

important aspect of Ayurveda and is what links up the cellular communication between the mind and the body. In yoga, the mode of sustaining life is through the operation of *prana*.

So, without metabolism, cell reproduction and intercellular communication, there is no life. This concept, therefore, gives us an insight into the importance of maintaining these systems – this is what Ayurveda and yoga aim to do. What we put into our bodies and how we do so is fundamental to the way we function. Being physically healthy gives us the opportunity to be more emotionally balanced, and the more emotionally balanced we are, the more physically in balance we are likely to be. Ultimately, physical and emotional balance leads to happiness, and the happier we become, the better able we are to connect to and fulfil our life's purpose – which, for the Indian mystics, was the whole point.

Without a balanced metabolism (*agni*), it is impossible to sustain a good state of health. For this we need the right balance of enzymes, hormones and neurotransmitters in order to fire the metabolism correctly. Getting this balance right can be tricky. Your body will have its own unique state of balance, or the ideal, balanced expression of your genetic makeup as discussed above. Some people, for example, may naturally metabolize slower than others and seek more nurturing activities in their balanced and free state, while others may naturally metabolize more quickly and seek high-paced activities. The more you become in tune with yourself, the more you will begin to understand what activities, tastes and meal quantities you enjoy and serve you well, leaving you feeling fit and vital – and

which ones are less suited to you. When we do not observe and listen, when we live a stressful lifestyle and fail to nourish ourselves properly on a daily basis, we are likely to propel ourselves further away from our own unique state of balance.

Additionally, we do not live in a sterile, controlled environment. Instead we live in a beautiful, ever-changing world, full of people that we connect with, and how we perceive and interpret this world around us, as well as how the world interacts with us, affects our balance. Ayurveda takes this into consideration and provides some wonderful tips on how to stay in balance with the changing seasons and climate, as well as how to develop our inner equanimity so that we can optimize our connection with the outer world. I will share some of this wisdom with you throughout this book.

Ama (metabolic waste)

If, over the course of time we have been living quite far removed from our *prakruti*, we are likely to have accumulated some *ama* or waste matter. This waste can be viewed in both a physical and psychological form. The word means 'sludge', referring to undigested food, emotions or experiences left over in our bodies and minds. In order to move towards a better state of health, this waste matter must be slowly removed.

Every time we eat on the go or when digestion is weak, our bodies produce *ama*. Since, according to Ayurveda, *ama* is the root-cause of many diseases, it is imperative to reduce *ama* and bring the body back into balance. The kitchen is where we start this process and ignite the digestive fire or *agni*.

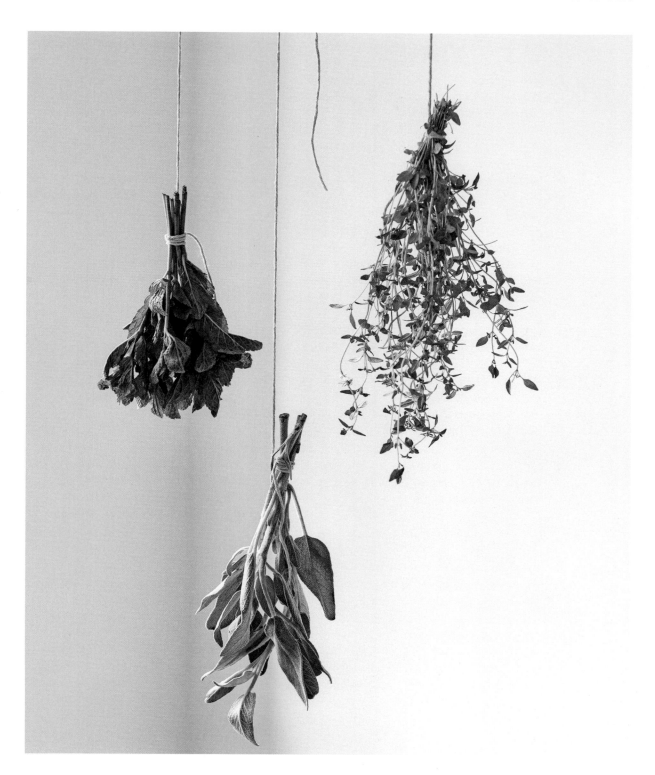

It is often a better idea to change patterns slowly rather than quickly, as this gives the body and mind adjustment time, preventing withdrawal symptoms. So, for example, if you currently drink between eight and ten cups of coffee or black tea per day, if you were to suddenly stop, there would be a likelihood of experiencing some uncomfortable physical symptoms for a short period of time. If, instead, you gradually cut down your intake and replace it with something like green tea (in which the caffeine interacts with the body in a completely different way and which additionally has many health benefits), the body slowly adjusts, misses the substance you are eradicating less and is less likely to experience withdrawal symptoms. If it is a habit you have been nurturing for 20 years, taking a few extra days or weeks to change it is no bad thing.

If your diet is currently very far from the types of food recommended in this book, you might like to dip your toe in gently and try out a couple of recipes and slowly incorporate this style of eating and way of being into your life. If you are more gung-ho and thrive on change, then do jump in and enjoy!

Some *ama* comes out of the system quite easily and you may find that some aches, pains and niggles recede as your system becomes clearer, but sometimes the backlog of sludge can be bigger, in which case you may need some herbal support. I have included a range of teas and a few recipes that can help to shift this unrequired *ama* (see Green Chai page 182, Honey and Trikatu Electuary page 87 or Cleansing Kitchari page 157).

When there have been unsupportive dietary practices in existence for a while, the range and levels of gut flora can be depleted. Good gut flora is essential for strong *agni* (digestive fire). Although we can repopulate our gut bacteria with foods, sometimes it can be hard to get a full range of strains into the gut, in which case you may need to supplement for a while. Eating regularly and in tune with the seasons helps to promote a strong digestive system and can remove or prevent *ama* accumulation.

Modern relevance

Humans have changed marginally, both physically and psychologically, since the inception of Ayurveda as a science, and much of the teachings and guiding principles of Ayurveda remain relevant today. Moreover, in a world where we have become disconnected in many senses from a more natural way of life, its teachings are possibly even more relevant now.

Ayurveda was designed to be a living science, not a fixed science, so we can adapt it to today's world and the changes that have come about in our species over the millennia. For example, the age of menstrual onset is earlier than it was and menopause is later, which has different metabolic implications for women. In this book, I interweave much of these age-old teachings into the fabric of our everyday lives to help us to regain and retain balance, as much as possible, while remaining open to current knowledge and science, and thus be able to thrive.

Having allowed myself to be influenced by modern science, today the way I treat clients is very different to the approach I took ten years ago, yet I would describe myself as being a traditional Ayurvedic practitioner both then and now. For instance, there has been an explosion in research into the gut microbiome, and this has helped to explain some of the importance Ayurveda places on good *agni* (digestive fire) and the role of the large intestine in good health. This has influenced my recommendations to clients to improve their digestive health. For instance, I often recommend some incredibly effective Ayurvedic probiotic formulations to address gut imbalances, whereas previously I would have sometimes relied on *Takra* formulations (buttermilk or yogurt mixed with spices).

A plant-based approach?

Much commentary is given in Ayurvedic texts as to the nature and medicinal properties of different types of meat and fish. Some people believe that this information is given purely for medicinal purposes and that, unless meat and fish are being used for these reasons, a vegetarian diet should be followed. I have no personal beliefs or views either way about meat and fish consumption. I have witnessed some clients benefit from reintroducing meat and fish into their diet, while others have benefitted from reducing their meat and fish consumption. What is important is that you establish your beliefs about the subject and then make your own choices in accordance with these beliefs. Along with this, if you are vegetarian or vegan, it is really important to supplement any dietary components that may be missing from your diet, such as calcium, vitamin D, vitamin B_{12}, iodine, selenium, zinc, iron and omega-3 fats.

As a general rule of thumb, if you choose to eat meat and fish and wish to add it to some of the recipes in this book, it is best to do this only a few times a week and to ensure that the it is well sourced. Keeping your total consumption low allows your body to digest the meat or fish from each meal well, which limits the burden that is placed on your body. Reducing your consumption also reduces the impact on the external environment. Meat should be well cooked, which helps to break down the fibres.

Healthy by design

Kitchens come in all shapes and sizes. By using the principles of Ayurveda and a little vision, you can turn any space into an Ayurveda Kitchen that nourishes body, mind and soul.

For millennia, humans have understood the value of laying out space in an aesthetically and energetically pleasing way. Our design principles take their guiding cues from the stunning structures found in nature. This can be seen in traditions such as the Ayurvedic form of *vastu* and the Chinese system of *feng shui*, for example. A well laid out kitchen can give rise to feelings of harmony, balance and endless possibilities for creativity and joy. This sets the scene for creating food that is nourishing and pleasing, and leads to a better state of health and wellbeing. By giving our kitchens the right kind of design input, we can create an environment pulsing with the essence of life or *prana*, uplifting our state of mental and physical wellness.

You do not need to have lots of space or money to establish your own Ayurveda Kitchen. When I was in India doing my internship, I created mine in the corner of my bedroom with a camping stove. My organization and the attitude I took to that space allowed me to create wholly nourishing meals that filled me with vitality and energy. In this section, I take you through the different factors to bear in mind when considering how to adjust your kitchen to make it more nurturing and pleasing to the senses.

Thoughtful layout

Although working with a clean slate can be fun, there is no need to completely redesign your kitchen to improve its layout. A few simple changes can go a long way towards making the space work better for you.

Consider utilizing the Japanese management concept of *kaizen*. *Kai* means 'change' and *zen* means 'good flow' or 'pleasing flow'. *Kaizen* is a concept of continually improving your processes to attain an optimum output. The idea here is to create an efficient layout in your kitchen so you can operate more productively within it. For instance, are your cooking utensils, cooking oils, seasonings and spices stored near to the stove? Anything you may need to hand when you are cooking should be as close to the cooker as possible, while items like crockery and silverware can be stored further away – ideally, close to the dining table. Spending time thinking about how to rearrange your kitchen will pay high dividends down the line. Take time to assess the layout critically and objectively.

Make it uplifting

We all have different tastes and styles and our homes offer an opportunity to express ourselves. For instance, some people thrive with bountiful colours on display, while others prefer subdued tones. There is no single perfect style, but there is a magic perfect design for *you*, to be created by *you*. By applying some general guiding principles (see box, page 24) you can cultivate a kitchen environment you feel nurtured by, in which you can create nourishing meals for yourself and your family and friends.

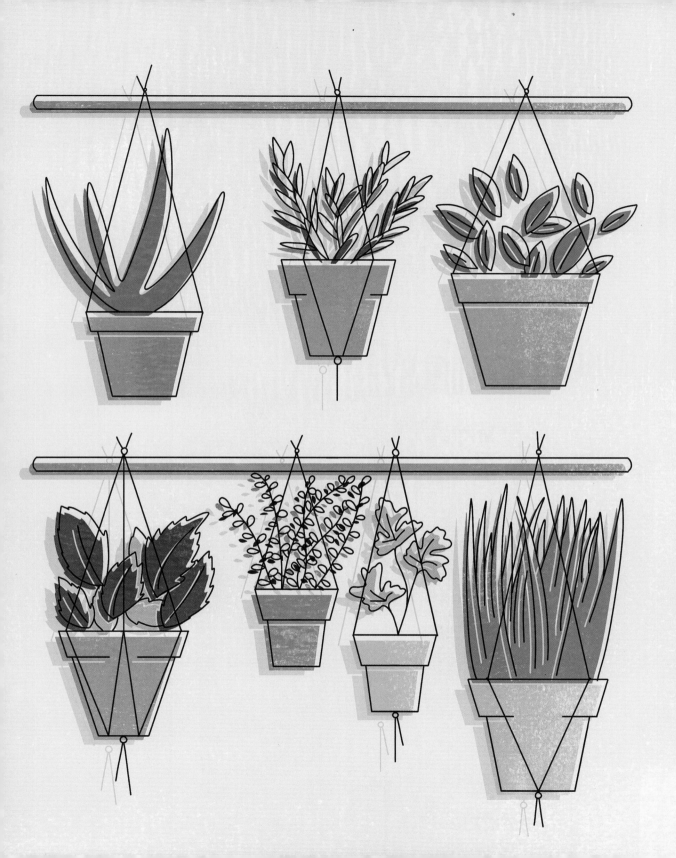

Uplifting your kitchen need not cost the earth or create more damage and waste for the environment. Below are a few ideas to get your creative juices flowing. Use local hardware shops as well as charity, vintage and antique shops, and also local thrift websites to obtain items you need to give your kitchen the facelift you are after.

Kitchen makeover tips

- When choosing paint colours, select those that give you a feeling of joy and make you want to live and thrive in the space. You are looking to create an environment that beckons to you and in which you feel safe, happy and refreshed.

- Lighting is something that can easily be adjusted and can make a huge difference to how you feel and operate in a space. Good lighting in a kitchen is important – it allows you to see well what you are cooking. It also allows your plants to thrive – plants grow well in artificial light, so do not worry if you cannot increase your natural lighting.

- Changing drawer handles and doorknobs is very easy to do and can give your kitchen a different feel instantly.

- Painting the fronts of your kitchen cupboards can revamp a tired old kitchen in a matter of hours. Look out for low-toxicity paints, which are better for you and better for the environment. Consider replacing flooring with natural materials, such as FSC wood, or man-made eco-friendly ones, such as Marmoleum.

- Are there items in your kitchen that could be relocated somewhere else in the house? For example, if your washing machine is in the kitchen, could it be moved to a cupboard, a utility room or a cloakroom?

- Introduce some life into your kitchen with pots of herbs or perhaps even a living wall of herbs. See pages 66–7 for ideas on nurturing plants in the kitchen.

- An inexpensive and quick way of enhancing your kitchen is to put up shelving on free wall space. This allows you to claim back countertop space from items that can be stored away on shelves in boxes or baskets. (Use the additional surface space for keeping plants.)

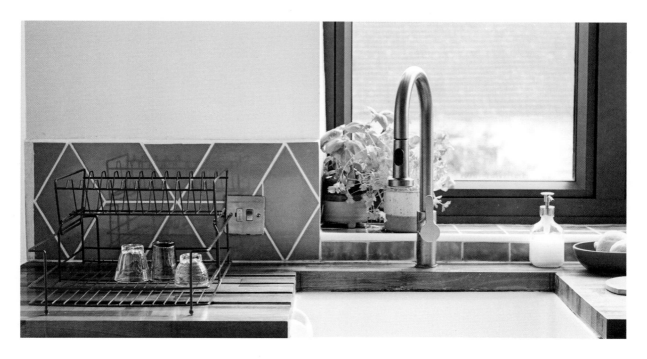

Minimize clutter

For some people, having a little clutter can give them a feeling of safety, while for others, it can drive them to distraction. Being the heart of the house, kitchens tend to serve as perfect dumping grounds for 'life stuff'. The old adage of 'tidy house, tidy mind' could not be more apt in the kitchen. Clutter takes up vital preparation space. There is always a wonderful feeling created when it is removed and space is regained. It somehow feels internally cleansing. However, it is also important to be realistic about what your clutter-gathering tendencies are, especially during busy times, when it is more challenging to find the time and energy to put things away properly. A simple solution is to have a clutter drawer that is periodically sorted through and emptied. If drawer space is at a premium, perhaps use a basket or a little chest that can be tucked away somewhere. The key thing is to get your clutter off the surfaces where possible.

Envisage your ideal space

With the guiding principles listed opposite in mind, try the following exercise. Close your eyes and imagine what your dream kitchen would look like. You can jot down a few notes.

Now step into your actual kitchen as if it is the first time you are seeing it. Look at it through the lens of your dream kitchen and establish what small and easy changes you can make to bring it closer to your dream.

Taking inspiration from the notes you have written, make a five-point action plan for what you can realistically do to work towards your goal. Initially, this may be some rearranging, deck clearing, decluttering or *prana* filling (increasing the presence of life energy and feeling of vitality in the space). Over time, you may be able to incorporate a larger layout and decorative adjustments that lead to significant changes in how nurtured you feel in the space.

Kitchen gadgets

We have all been tempted with every kind of kitchen gadget imaginable. However, I encourage you to explore the idea that less is more. Now is the time to discern what equipment is actually needed to make wholesome food – which, in truth, is very little.

The more equipment we fill our kitchens with, the fewer opportunities we have to connect with the raw ingredients we are preparing, and the less we experience a sense of satisfaction in the end product. Electrical equipment also tends to be bulky and can take up valuable space that can otherwise be allocated to growing *prana*-giving plants and sprouts (see pages 66 and 68).

Kitchen gadgets generally perform repetitive tasks, but bear in mind that performing these tasks yourself can be wholly supportive of both mental and physical health. A lot of the benefit gained through the practice of yoga is from the repetitive nature of many postures, along with pure mindful focus and the engagement of both sides of the body. This same mindset can be brought into the kitchen, especially with more repetitive physical tasks, such as whisking, shredding, grating and kneading. It is all a question of cooking with consciousness – with attention and connection, and with focus on your intention (see pages 36–8).

Having said all this, the obvious advantage of kitchen equipment is that it can help to save time. If you are desperately time poor and, by using some kit, you are able and inspired to make nutritious food, then of course it would be ridiculous to not use it to your advantage. You can still consciously set your intention and inner attitude and be mindful of your posture.

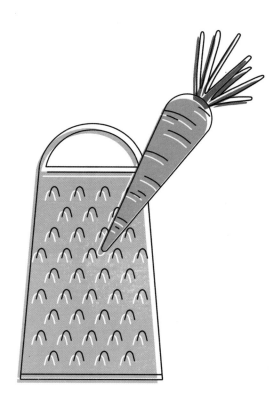

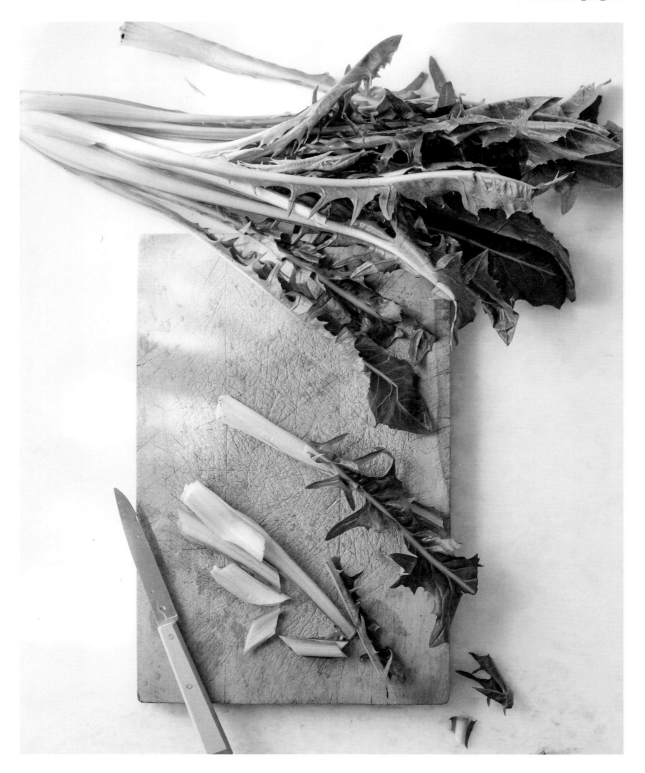

Stocking your kitchen _____

Running an Ayurveda Kitchen offers the opportunity to bring a higher level of conscious thought to how we stock it. Our shopping habits put pressure on suppliers to make better environmental choices, so use your purchasing power wisely.

In many parts of the world today, we can obtain any food from any corner of the globe very easily, but this comes at a huge environmental cost. In order to get these foods to us they often have a high carbon footprint, they are heavily packaged to protect them in transit and natural environments are often ruthlessly destroyed to create growing conditions for them.

According to Ayurveda, the most suitable foods and herbs are those that are grown locally to the person consuming them (see below). The reason for this is that they contain the microbiota and qualities that are most suited to the individual in that given season. Eating locally like this requires some effort though, and for those who live in metropolitan areas it may be impractical. But we might make a few small changes to eat more seasonally and locally, and reduce the amount of foods we buy in plastic packaging.

Order in bulk

Stocking a kitchen well drives our inspiration to cook. If you open your cupboards or look on your shelves and see a range of dried ingredients, this can give you a desire to get the saucepans out, as well as an inner feeling of abundance. There is an environmental gain too – it is more cost effective, carbon efficient and minimizes packaging when you order in bulk. The only drawback with bulk ordering

can be storage requirements. If your storage space is limited, you may need to source your food more frequently in order to keep stocks up.

Buy local

Look at where the food you are buying has travelled from. Ingredients such as cashew nuts, rice and coconut all have high food miles associated with them. By keeping your diet varied, seasonal and local, you cut your food miles dramatically. That is not to say that you should not enjoy some treats from faraway shores once in a while. Being an Ayurvedic practitioner, trained in the use of ingredients that originate in the Indian subcontinent, I have had to think carefully about many of the foods and herbs I use. For me, finding local alternatives with the desired qualities is key to generating a sustainable practice.

Buying locally can also make it easier to obtain fruit and vegetables that are free of packaging. Generally, fruit-and-veg box schemes deliver without any plastics being used and are a simple solution if you are short of time. Using local markets to buy fruit and vegetables is another easy way to avoid packaging. It can be done in supermarkets too, but you might need to take some paper/cotton bags with you, or be prepared to manage your apples rolling around.

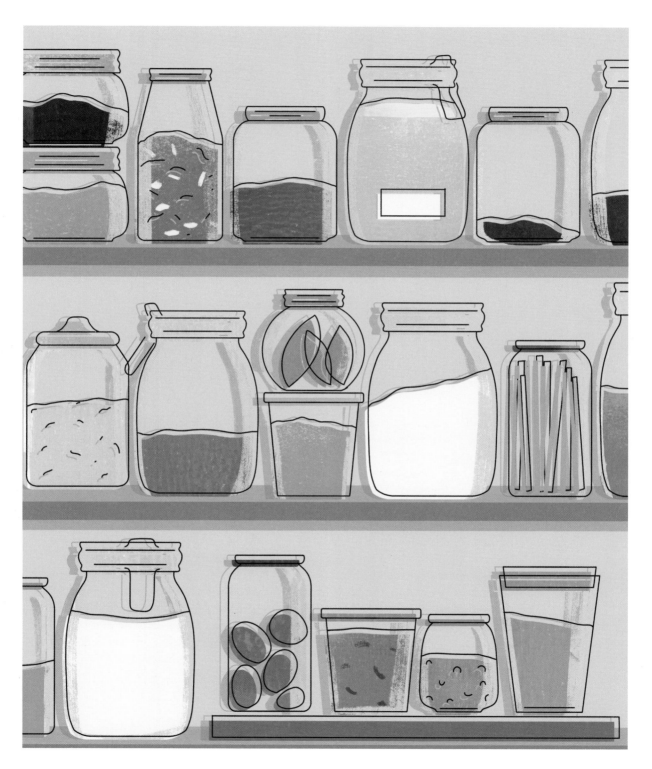

Buying dry goods in bulk and either in plant-based packaging or in our own reusable packaging reduces our personal carbon footprint and reduces waste.

Stick to fresh

Processed foods are often less nourishing than unprocessed foods and are invariably heavily packaged. By reducing processed items, you can create wholesome food to support yourself physically and mentally while reducing waste production.

Storage tips

- Utilize large glass storage jars to keep dried goods fresh for longer periods of time and stop pests from intruding. Label the contents so you know what they are.

- Keep dried herbs and spices in the dark, ideally in a cupboard or drawer. They lose their potency after varying amounts of time, so monitor your stocks well. Always smell them – they should give off a good aroma, even before cooking with them, and look vibrant. The older they become, the more you will be missing out on their digestion-enhancing and medicinal qualities. Buying large bulk quantities of your go-to herbs and less of the others ensures good rotation. Do not be afraid to put old herbs you have not touched for years into the compost bin and start again.

- Understand which foods are best kept in the refrigerator and which are better suited to a cool, dark cupboard. For example, tomatoes are better off on the countertop to enhance their ripening process and sweet taste. Pumpkins and squashes, on the other hand, love to sit in a cool, dark place for a couple of months, which enhances their unique properties.

Cleaning your kitchen _____

How you clean is important. It is not just a matter of good hygiene – appropriate cleaning makes the kitchen feel loved and cared for. We all instinctively gravitate towards spaces we feel offer us trust, safety and shelter – this is the concept underlying the Ayurveda Kitchen and cleanliness underpins it.

Keeping a kitchen clean can be a ritual that serves you in its own right. Rather than seeing it as a chore, it is an opportunity to create balance and beauty, and increase the vibrancy of your space. It is also an opportunity to create balance in your body. When we clean we tend to engage our dominant side. Try wiping surfaces or washing one or two pots with your opposite hand. This might feel a little awkward to begin with, but as time progresses it will become easier. These are great exercises for the brain, creating new neural pathways.

Cleaning products

What you choose to clean your kitchen with is important. Using low-toxicity products is preferable – they are better for both you and the environment. By making this choice you are actively practising the yogic concept of *ahimsa* (non-violence) towards yourself and all of nature, especially aquatic life.

Classically in Ayurveda, herbs such as strong-smelling neem (highly anti-bacterial) and cows' urine (which has a high ammonia content) were predominately used as cleaning agents, and cow dung was burnt to purify the atmosphere in a practice known as *agnihotra*, but I am not suggesting you use these methods. Instead, try making the cleaning products on page 33.

There is a whole world to be discovered in making your own cleaning products. Once you get started, you might want to experiment. If so, bear in mind that the acidic nature of vinegar or the very alkali nature of bicarbonate of soda makes them unsuitable for some work tops. They are best suited to ceramics, glass, man-made tiles and stainless steel. So, they are great to clean toilets and bathrooms, but not natural stone, for which Castile soap is better. Castile soap can, in fact, be used on all types of surfaces.

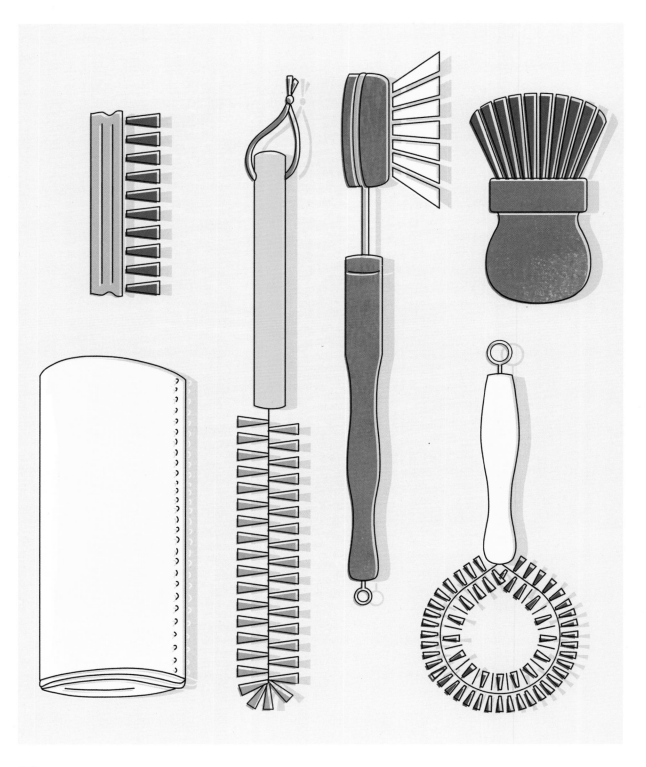

Glass-cleaning spray

This mixture does an excellent job of sprucing up and de-smearing glass. The product will not keep for very long once mixed, so you may want to mix up as much as you need for a week or so at a time.

200ml (⅓ pint) filtered water
50ml (2fl oz) white vinegar

Mix the water and vinegar together and store in an upcycled spray bottle, ready for use. Use a glass-cleaning or lint-free cloth when cleaning.

Clearing the air

Use the soothing aromas of essential oils to lift the atmosphere in your Ayurveda Kitchen. Essential oil burners or diffusers are relatively inexpensive, and enable you to make use of the healing properties of essential oils. Add three drops of your chosen essential oil to some water to purify the air and support your needs. For instance, use: eucalyptus essential oil when feeling congested physically, mentally or emotionally; lavender essential oil if feeling stressed or anxious; or camphor oil when in need of some vitality.

Sink cleaner

Ensure you wear a pair of gloves when using this mixture, which can also be used to clean your toilets.

2 tablespoons bicarbonate of soda
2 tablespoons white vinegar
squeeze of lemon juice

Close the sink plug hole with a plug. Put the bicarbonate of soda in the sink, followed by the vinegar and lemon juice. At first it will fizz, then it will settle. Leave for around 5 minutes, then scrub the sink with a brush. Now open the plug hole and turn on the hot tap to wash away the bicarbonate of soda and vinegar. The added advantage to using this product is that it will clean your drains too.

Surface-cleaning spray

2 tablespoons Castile soap
200ml (⅓ pint) filtered water
10 drops tea tree essential oil
5 drops lavender essential oil

Mix the ingredients together and store in an upcycled spray bottle, ready for use. Spray the product onto your kitchen surfaces and leave for a few moments before wiping off with a wet linen cloth.

Invite consciousness _____

You can bring spirit and energy into your kitchen through conscious thought and mindful experience. A great way of doing this is to engage the senses when in the space.

By engaging your senses as part of your kitchen experience, the room becomes less of a mechanistic space that simply produces fuel, and more of a vital living space that inspires you to create delicious meals, which are going to nourish you.

The way you think about your kitchen informs the way you operate within it. The more you consciously think about it as a healing space, offering potential for vitality and fulfilment, the more likely it is that it becomes that for you. Below I suggest ways in which you can explore this concept through your five senses, as this is how we experience the world.

Sight

By visually stimulating and refreshing the look of your kitchen, you are instantly bringing fresh energy to the space. If you then continue to tend to the look of your kitchen, this helps to give it a feeling of life. Consciously bringing in plants instantly gives it a visual vibrancy.

Sound

The sounds you generate from cooking animate the space. From time to time bring your attention to the sound of bubbles from boiling pans of water and pans being stirred, or the tinkling of whisks hitting bowls. These sounds may often pass us by, but they are an intrinsic part of cooking and something that can be paid attention to. Bringing our awareness to these sounds deepens our connection with the cooking process and can have a positive mental-health benefit as part of a mindful practice.

Smell

Aroma is paramount to good cooking and good flavour. What we are actually looking for in terms of a base smell in a kitchen is one of neutrality – a clean-smelling plain canvas onto which we paint our myriad of culinary scents. The cooking smells then build up, which contributes to creating a memory associated with the kitchen space. The more layers of aromas we create, the more we reinforce this notion that the kitchen is a living space, and we feel inwardly motivated to be in it and create nourishment for ourselves. The aromas we create tickle our gustatory system, sending biochemical messages around the body and priming our digestive system to receive our lovingly prepared food with gratitude.

Touch

The majority of us who are gifted with sight tend to over-rely on it. Have you ever felt your way around your kitchen? It can be a fun, insightful and humbling exercise. Bringing a little conscious awareness to the way your kitchen feels can give you a new experience of your environment. Caressing the leaves of your pot herbs, running your fingers over your freshly cleaned countertops or really feeling the running water from your kitchen tap can generate a more enriched experience of your kitchen. Touch is a sense that can be brought out when cleaning or handling vegetables and when performing any kind of kneading activity.

Taste

The taste of the kitchen is really in its aromas – and then in the food, of course. The more vibrant the aromas, the tastier the food will be, and the more people entering your home will literally be able to sense that in the air.

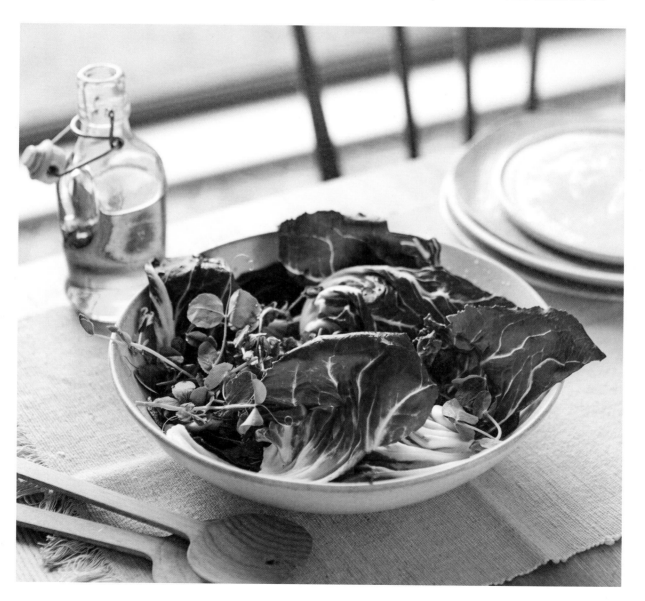

Cooking with consciousness _____

I believe that when we bring the attitude and intention of love towards our cooking something softens and flavours somehow develop more fully. According to Ayurveda, the energy of the chef is imparted to the meal they make, so bring your full and loving attention to food preparation to add to its health-giving properties.

The kitchen is a wonderful place to practise mindfulness. Being in the present moment has enormous health benefits to your mental and physical health. In energetic terms, it also benefits anyone who eats the meals you prepare. So start to look upon the act of cooking as a meditative task and give it your full attention.

Set your intention

To bring a sense of reverence to the process of cooking, begin each time by defining and setting your intention. When making a cake, for instance, start by setting your intention at the outset. This might be to create a wholesome, delicious, well-risen cake that is going to bring much pleasure to you in the baking process. Or perhaps through the baking process you would like to feel more relaxed at the end and connected to the world around you. See if you can start to develop a feeling of connection between you, the abundance of the ingredients, your involvement in this process of baking and the sense of achievement you will have at the end of it, irrespective of how it turns out.

Mindful attention

When you begin the work, bring your mindful attention to the process. For instance, if you are chopping a carrot, give the act your full focus. (This has the added benefit of you being less likely to lose the end of a finger.)

If your mind wanders off, simply bring it back to the process, as you would if you were meditating.

When we are able to give any given task our full attention, the end result is usually much better than when we are distracted. Therefore, the food you have prepared is likely to be tastier, more akin to what you were aiming to produce, and you are able to listen to any inner dialogue that will help you to modify your cooking to suit your current state. (For example, if you are not distracted, your inner voice might tell you, 'I am feeling cold right now and could do with a little more paprika in the dish today.')

Life in a full and busy household, however, does not always allow you to give food preparation your full, unadulterated attention, so we accept the situation, do what we can and maintain an inner feeling of focus and bring love to the multitasking. This acceptance and development of inner feelings becomes another form of mindfulness.

What we think about food is as important as what we actually eat. If we connect mindfully with the food we are cooking and think about it from this stage onwards as being health-giving and balancing then, in Ayurveda, we believe that this will become a reality for us.

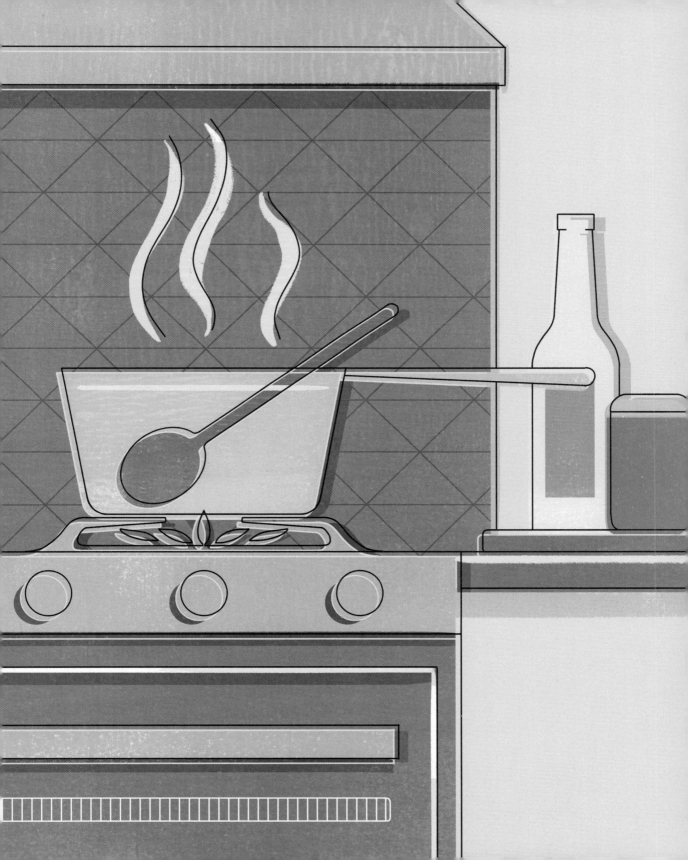

Any mindful activity supports our mental health by creating mental space and encouraging mental harmony. Mindful kitchen activities are aimed at bringing harmony by tying together the action of the senses with thought process and bodily activities. This tying together can bring an inner feeling of calm and be very grounding in its nature. In Ayurveda and yoga, we consider this to be a *sattvic* (harmonious) way of being.

Postural awareness

As you work, be aware of your posture. Are you standing with your weight evenly distributed? Do you need to drop your shoulders? Do you need to take your breath deeper and allow it to become slower? Cooking is a wonderful opportunity to address physical imbalances. For instance, when chopping a carrot, notice if you have engaged any unnecessary parts of your body in the process – perhaps your facial muscles and jaw have tightened? Whatever you notice is going on with you, you can decide to make a change consciously, readjust your posture and engage only the muscles that are needed for the task.

Tasks such as whisking and stirring offer a great opportunity to balance out our left and right sides. Most of us tend to favour using our dominant side, causing physical misalignment, with certain muscle groups on one side of the body becoming stronger than those on the other side. This ultimately puts pressure on the joints. The kitchen is a the perfect place to even out this favouritism. Whenever you are stirring or whisking, first plant your feet into the ground, grow tall out of your feet and assess if your weight is distributed evenly across both feet. Then, if you are right handed, deliberately take the spoon or whisk in your left hand and give it a turn for as long as is comfortable for you. Just before your hand begins to tire, switch back to your right hand, maintaining even weight distribution between both feet throughout. If you are stirring or whisking for a long time, keep switching from side to side.

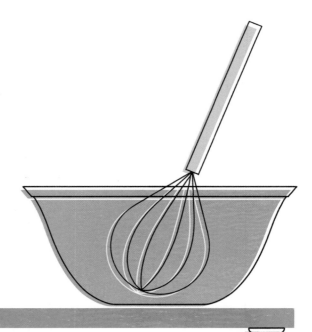

Dining with consciousness _____

When, where and how you eat will all have an effect on how well your digestive system processes the food you consume. Eating mindfully will greatly improve the effectiveness of your metabolism.

When to eat

In Ayurveda, balanced mealtimes are vital to creating digestive harmony within the body. The intention is to try to consume three meals a day. Let your energy and environment inform the size of your portions. In winter, or if you have been working hard, you may find you may need to eat more. Timings of meals are important. We are creatures that run on an internal clock and our metabolic system is closely tied to sunlight through our circadian rhythms. Eating daily at roughly 7am, 12.30pm and 6pm gives huge benefit. Ideally, you should not eat after 8pm. If you work night shifts, then the meal times should be kept regular and nourishing throughout the night. By eating good foods at the right times, a true hunger-driven need for a snack is unlikely to appear. If, however, you have been working hard physically, a small snack may be required.

Where to eat

Where you eat your lovingly prepared meals is of importance. As a general guide, Ayurveda advises eating in a quiet, soothing environment. I have seen huge amounts of positive change in clients who have merely adjusted when and how they eat. An optimum mealtime would involve you sitting down at a table with both feet placed on the floor and a neutral spine, or sitting on your heels on the floor with your food on something that resembles a low table. These postures do not create any twists and turns in the plumbing pipework that comprises our digestive system.

How to eat

You may have cooked your meal mindfully, but it is important to eat it mindfully as well. Give your full focus to your meal and the act of eating. We are psychological and physiological beings – the more we are mentally engaged in something other than eating, the more other systems are triggered by our brains and the less effective our metabolic system will be at processing our meal. So, in plain English, this means no screens, no books and no intense thinking about projects or work.

Before you take your first bite, take a brief moment to connect with the food in front of you. Look at it, smell it and express some inner gratitude for it (see page 40). The smelling stage is very important. Fragrant foods release phenols, flavour compounds that trigger the sense of smell and tell the brain to prepare for food. This further initiates a wave of enzyme activity as the body prepares to receive the forthcoming bounty.

The first bite is always the best bite for me, but for the entire meal, try to be aware of the different textures in your mouth. Take time to chew your food. Not only does this break down the food particles efficiently, leaving less of a burden for the rest of our digestive system, but the act of chewing also actually stimulates a host of digestive processes. If you can, avoid excessive talking or laughing while eating – the less air you take in along with your food, the less chance there is of hiccups, abdominal discomfort and belching after you have finished.

Stop when you are full. By eating more consciously you are likely to be able to sense more readily when you have reached your natural capacity. Our food intake requirements change constantly, according to our energy output, environmental factors including the weather and fluctuating emotional states. The more connected to ourselves we become, the more understanding we can be of our digestive needs. This will then affect our own inner portion control.

The importance of gratitude

We rarely stop to think about how food connects us to thousands of other people whom we have never met before, who have collaborated to bring the food to our plates. Then think about the millions of bacteria, insects and animals that are likely to have played their part. There is much to be grateful for. Acknowledgement should also go to yourself, for taking the time to prepare the meal for yourself and possibly others with love. By expressing gratitude, you can stimulate a more glass-half-full-style mental state, which in turn stimulates a positive psychosomatic feedback loop within the body. All of this means that our body's 'digestive fire' (see page 18) is more ready to convert and devour the diverse range of life-giving materials we are supplying it with.

Take a moment before you start your meal to express some thanks for the food. This can be as simple as a few thoughts, or formulated and even ritualized as a prayer, if that resonates with you. You could do this either in your mind or out loud, if you feel comfortable, and do share it, if that works for you. I like to say internally the following: 'I express heartfelt thanks for the wonderful meal before me. May it create balance within me and be well digested and processed, leaving me feeling satisfied and nourished.'

Reality bites

Sometimes we have little choice in the nature of the environment in which we find ourselves at mealtimes, and it may seem as though time limits or stressful situations hamper our best attempts at eating with consciousness. Nevertheless, challenging situations do not need to trigger a stress response and result in impaired digestion. The more we can cultivate inner peace and harmony, the less likely these external situations are to influence our stress response. The more relaxed and content you can be, the better able you will be to digest your food and the more you will benefit from the ingredients and all their heavenly constituents.

The last thing I want you to do though, is to create more stress by bringing the focus too much on 'trying to relax'. That would be counterproductive. It is important that you connect with an inward motivation to change and work with yourself with loving kindness, not against yourself.

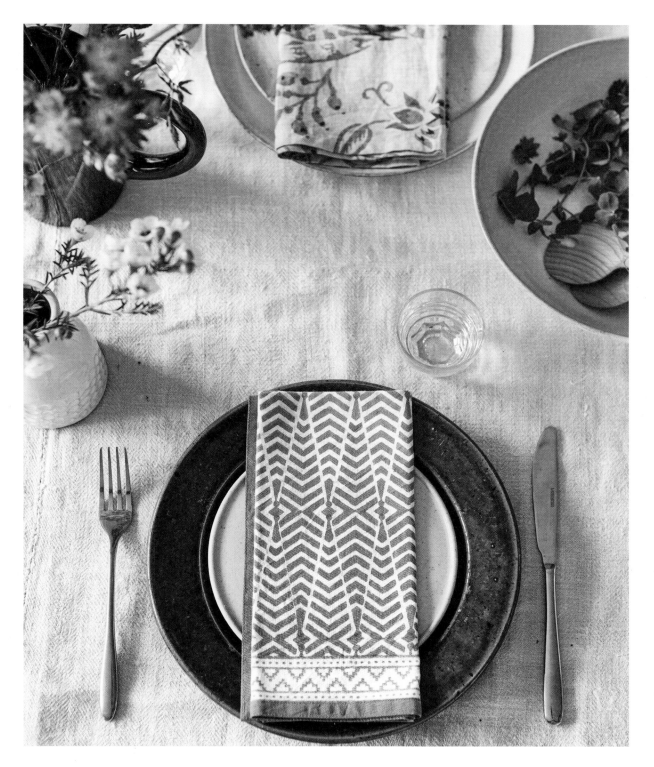

Tricky mealtime tips

Below is some practical advice suggesting things you can do to practise mindful eating within challenging situations. Even if your own circumstances are not precisely represented here, the approaches described may still be of use to you.

Busy lunch
You have cooked yourself a delicious packed lunch to take to work with you. The morning has been intense, with lots of appointments. You were hungry at 12.30pm but it is now 1.30pm and you have only just found time to eat. There is nowhere obvious to eat lunch, but you manage to find a quiet corner of the building where you can stand and have 10 minutes to yourself. The tendency here might be to just dive straight in as you are so hungry and your thoughts are already rushing to what you have coming up in the afternoon. Equally, you might be tempted to read a few emails or respond to a few texts while you eat.

This is where a little self-discipline is required, which will pay dividends later in the afternoon. Firstly, simply, stop. Stand still, readjust your posture and let your breathing rate normalize. Allow a couple of elongated conscious breaths to roll in and out. This will take no more than a minute, but will help you focus on eating, not the external work environment. Open up your packed lunch and inhale the smell of the food. This is a vital step as it immediately sets in motion a cascade of digestive secretions. Take the first bite and really taste the food. When we are rushed, food can barely touch the insides of our

mouths, which are densely packed with taste receptors that need to be hit to stimulate digestion. Then, mouthful by mouthful, enjoy each morsel of the food. When you have finished, take a brief moment to acknowledge the nourishment you have just gifted yourself. This will initiate a feeling of love for yourself, which is hugely powerful, especially during a busy day.

Challenging home life
Your home life is currently emotionally challenging. Mealtimes are fraught with tension, leading to physical tension within the digestive system as well.

Options are limited here – being creative and playful within your own head is sometimes all that is available. Take a few gentle breaths, focusing on the meal in front of you instead of the chaos around you, and connect with your food. We have complete access to our own inner thoughts and feelings, which the outside world need not be aware of, so if you find yourself in a miserable mealtime setting, play internally with visualizing and imagining a different setting. See if it helps bring a calmer inner feeling to you and thus aids your digestion. Perhaps one day you will be graced with a more pleasurable external setting that will require less effort to enjoy fully the bountiful meal you have lovingly created.

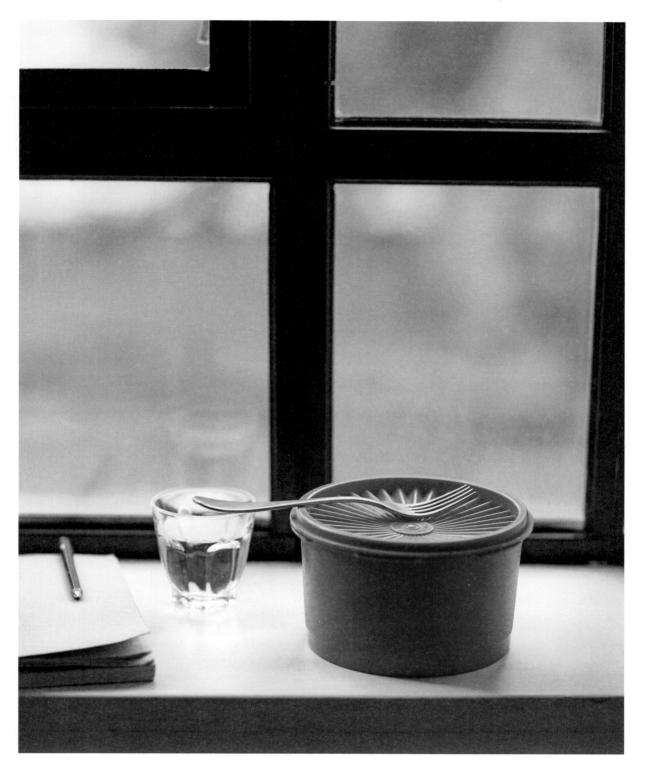

The breath and digestion _____

Quite incredibly, how we breathe can affect our sense of taste, appetite and digestive efficiency. Irrespective of what type of food you are eating, to have the optimal chance of digesting it well, an efficient and effective breathing technique is essential.

A relaxed diaphragmatic breathing style (see below) creates a feeling of relaxation. Slow breathing activates the parasympathetic nervous system, which creates homeostasis (equilibrium) in the body and promotes digestion, absorption and excretion.

Conversely, long-term stress leads to an increase in adrenaline release, heart rate and blood pressure and acidity pH levels within the stomach as the body's flight-or-fight reflex is triggered. During stressful periods, breathing patterns can become erratic and we fall into a cycle of chest breathing, in which shallow breaths are drawn in using the chest cavity only. When we use only our chest cavity to breathe, our digestive system misses out on a lot of the lovely massage it receives when we use the diaphragm to breathe. This massage is important when it comes to good digestion, both mechanically and chemically.

Diaphragmatic breathing

Relaxed diaphragmatic breathing improves your ability to cope in difficult situations and minimizes the chances of increases in stomach acidity levels. This means that, when it comes to meal times, there is a greater chance that the right pH level will be present to digest food properly, leading to more post-eating digestive comfort. It causes proper rhythmic movement further down the torso, positively affecting the organs all the

way down to the bladder. The whole of our musculature moves inwards and outwards when we breathe properly, creating a ripple effect over these organs.

This style of breathing is known as 'diaphragmatic', because the diaphragm moves downwards within the body as you inhale, enlarging the space available for the lungs to expand into as they fill with air. You know if you are breathing in this way if your chest, ribcage and belly expand outwards when you inhale. As you slowly inhale, draw the breath down towards the belly. Your ribcage should expand in all directions – forwards, sideways and backwards. The air continues to fill the chest cavity so that the chest lifts upwards. Reverse the process through the nose on the exhalation, allowing the belly, ribcage and chest to retract.

You may find initially that your ribcage does not move much but, after a few breaths, you may be able to feel it moving more as it becomes more engaged in the process. The inhalations and exhalations need to be done in a relaxed fashion, allowing an expansion of the ribcage. I have deliberately suggested here to 'relax and allow' the expansion rather than drive it, as you might with exercise. There is a good reason for this. Quite often, poor breathing techniques are initiated during periods of stress, and the last thing that is desired here is to initiate further mechanical stress and release of stress hormones in the body.

Once you are comfortable with the technique, enhance the experience by creating a mental image alongside the physical practice. As you gently allow the breath to roll in through the nose, the chest and towards the belly, with your eyes closed, try to create a mental image of the breath. You could picture it as a colour, a light, with a swirling quality – whatever image appeals most to you.

Whenever you are in your kitchen, bring your awareness to your breath to assess its depth. If you find your breaths are shallow, consciously practise diaphragmatic breathing. Before long, simply being in the kitchen will trigger your memory and you might automatically begin to breathe diaphragmatically each time you enter the space.

Breathing while eating

How you breathe while you are eating will also have an impact on your digestion. Allow no more than the necessary breath to be drawn in while eating. When food is consumed in a hurry, a lot of additional air can be drawn in too. This leads to indigestion and discomfort, which will present uncomfortably later on.

Eating well and breathing correctly bring about a metabolism that works as it should. When the metabolic and communication systems – or *agni* and *prana* (digestive fire and life force – see page 18) are functioning optimally, a good state of health is easier to achieve and maintain. Of course, life is not perfect. Sometimes the reason the metabolic system does not function perfectly is due to a genetic condition, acute illness or long-standing history of traumatic events. But even under these circumstances, eating well and breathing correctly can still help.

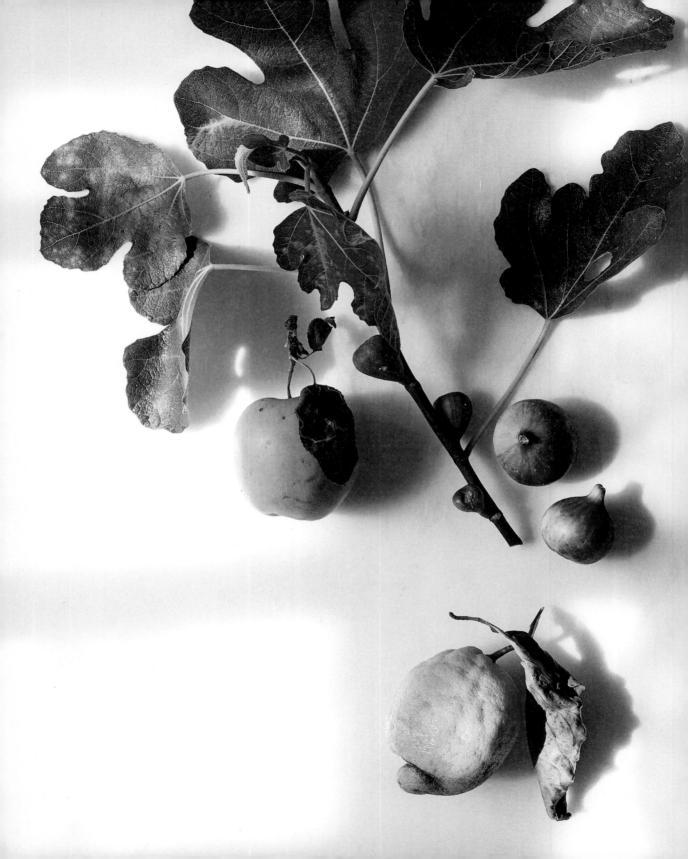

Ayurveda and seasonal eating

The six tastes _____

Ayurveda defines six categories of taste as the palate from which all foods draw their colourful flavours. The magic of Ayurvedic cooking lies in how seasonal ingredients are combined with the presence of all of the six tastes on the plate.

The six *rasas* (tastes)

In Ayurveda there are six tastes (see table opposite), and all foods fall into one or more of these flavour categories: sweet, sour, salty, bitter, pungent and astringent.

Balancing the tastes

When cooking, we are aiming to balance all six tastes in one meal, also paying consideration to your personal and seasonal preferences. The great thing about combining tastes is that one will inherently balance another. For instance, if you combine a very pungent and heating ingredient with something sweet and cooling, the resulting flavour will be completely different and one that is far more balanced. This type of combining is common in, say, Thai-style curries, in which hot chillies are combined with cooling coconut.

This balancing act is performed not only with the flavours of the ingredients in mind, but also with consideration of their medicinal properties. All foods are characterized not only by the taste categories they fall under, but also by whether they have a heating or cooling effect, and by their medicinal qualities.

Some of the magic of Ayurveda is its unique understanding of how things work in combination, some of which is now explained through science. For example, take a humble piece of broccoli. Alone it is primarily astringent in taste, also mildly bitter-sweet, and is cooling. If it is combined with mustard seeds, which are pungent and heating, this largely balances out the tastes. Some additional sour and salt can be added for full balance. It has recently been shown

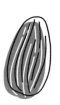
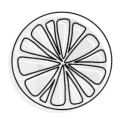
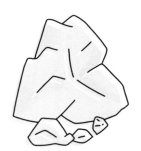
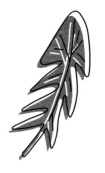
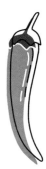
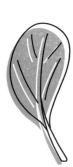

The *rasas*

Taste	Example	Role	Description
Sweet	Dates, sugar, milk	Promotes enzyme and pancreatic activity	The sweet taste is nourishing to all aspects of the body and is usually quite high in minerals. Sweet foods are comparatively hard to digest, but are very grounding, as this taste is made up of earth and water elements and is generally cold, oily and heavy.
Sour	Vinegar, lemon	Promotes stomach acid	The sour taste stimulates *agni* (see page 18). It often has high antioxidant activity. It is made of earth and fire and is generally hot, light and oily.
Salty	Sea salt, rock salt	Stimulates salivation by enhancing other flavours	The salty taste breaks down mucus and increases digestive activity. It is made of water and fire and is hot, oily and heavy.
Bitter	Chicory, dandelion greens	Promotes bile secretion	The bitter taste promotes liver and other digestive functions. It is often associated with cancer prevention due to its high levels of isothiocyanates, which are one of the bitter tasting principles. It is made of air and ether and is cold, light and dry.
Pungent	Black pepper, chilli	Increases blood flow by causing dilation of vessels	The pungent taste creates a tingling sensation on the tongue. It contributes to maintaining a healthy weight and can be used to treat obesity. It is made of fire and air and is hot, light and dry.
Astringent	Black tea, spinach, cranberries, red wine	Promotes water absorption, cleanses mucous membranes	The astringent taste creates a puckering feeling inside your cheeks. It is high in polyphenols, causing strong anti-microbial activity. It is made of air and earth and is cold and dry.

that adding mustard seeds at the end of cooking broccoli reintroduces an enzyme called myrosinase, which is lost during the cooking process of broccoli. This important enzyme unlocks some of the researched cancer-preventative properties of broccoli.

The chart opposite lists common ingredients and their tastes, and indicates whether their character is heating or cooling. Use this to help perform your own balancing act. I have chosen not to go into huge detail about which ingredients have which properties, listing only those that are likely to be used most often. Instead I have done the balancing job for you in the recipes in this book, giving you clues in each recipe as to how the ingredients have been balanced. My hope is that, through cooking the recipes, you will be able to learn how to create your own versions in your own style.

When it comes to choosing what you are going to cook, I find engaging your senses is helpful. Touch, feel and smell different ingredients and sense what moves you on a given day, then incorporate those ingredients into a meal.

Working with the seasons

Once you get a feel for the six tastes you can start to decide for yourself what you feel like combining on a given day. In Ayurveda we like to eat as closely as possible to what is growing in that particular season, to respond appropriately to climatic conditions. We prefer to eat warm, nourishing foods on cold days and cooler, more hydrating foods on hotter days. For example, if it is freezing cold outside, we need to cook using ingredients with opposite qualities (grounding, unctuous,

warming and calorifically sustaining). These qualities, by no accident, are in the foods that are seasonally available. By cooking with these things in mind we are showing love to ourselves and this, in turn, brings an inner feeling of harmony and relaxation.

Finally, you need to consider where you are at in all of this. If you have been emotionally challenged recently, you may be looking for food that gives you a feeling of comfort and love using your favourite ingredients. If, on the other hand, you have been enjoying a period of excess, you may need to lighten up the ingredients and trim down portion sizes. The more you begin to listen to your body and understand the food for yourself, the more you will be able to make these judgements of balance.

With these considerations in mind, you can start to work out what your individual tastes and needs are on a given day and work out what you want to add to the pot.

Key

- **Blue: Winter**

- **Green: Spring**

- **Yellow: Summer**

- **Brown: Autumn**

	Sweet	Sour	Salty	Bitter	Pungent	Astringent	Heating/Cooling
Beetroot	●			●			H
Brussel Sprout				●		●	H
Celeriac	●			●	●	●	H
Kale				●		●	C
Parsnip	●					●	C
Potato	●					●	C
Swede	●				●	●	H
Chestnut	●					●	H
Apple	●	●				●	C
Pear	●					●	C
Asparagus	●					●	C
New potato	●					●	C
Purple sprouting broccoli	●			●		●	C
Radish					●		H
Spinach		●				●	H
Spring onion					●		H
Watercress				●	●		H
Dandelion greens				●			H
Sorrel		●			●	●	H
Rhubarb		●					H
Artichoke	●					●	H
Broad / Runner / French beans	●					●	C
Courgette	●					●	C
Cucumber	●						C
Lettuce	●			●		●	C
Tomato	●	●					H
Mint	●				●		C
Peach	●	●				●	H
Melon	●						C
Strawberry	●	●				●	C
Aubergine				●		●	H
Broccoli	●			●		●	C
Butternut squash	●					●	C
Carrot	●						H
Cauliflower						●	C
Jerusalem artichoke				●		●	C
Pumpkin	●					●	C
Sweetcorn	●					●	H
Hazelnut						●	H
Blackberry	●	●				●	C
Fig	●						C

Seasonal kitchen *sadhana*

Sadhana is a term used to describe a daily practice that is done with a devotional and loving attitude. The idea behind the seasonal kitchen *sadhana* is the creation of a devotional practice in the kitchen that is informed by the attributes of the season.

At the change of each season, it is good to take a few hours to clean and prepare for the next season, clearing out any stale, left-over or processed foods to make room for more lively, vibrant foods that are full of life energy. We can ask ourselves what we feel we need in the new season, make delicious spice blends appropriate for the new season's fresh ingredients and create seasonal recipes to use in the coming weeks. These practical, mindful, nourishing acts help us create space in our lives for eating well.

By working with the different energy of the different seasons, it can be easier to find inner motivation for your activities. As we watch animals respond to the changes of the seasons we can start to understand how we should move with them too. Ayurveda classically describes six seasons but, today, we experience and classify only four, and I will focus on those four seasons here. Nature provides exactly the right types of food for us in each season, foods that nourish us and help to keep us in balance. By harvesting and preparing foods for storage throughout the growing season we are able to supplement what is not available. Ayurveda understands that certain foods actually increase in medicinal potency through storage – it is said that you can store ghee for one hundred years, for example. I have never managed more than about six months myself!

Use the guidelines in this section to move through the seasons with balance and grace.

Seasonal reset ritual

Consider performing the following ritual at home. Set aside 3 days in your calendar when you can take a break from your normal routine, preferably at the junction between seasons. In the days leading up to these three days, lighten your diet, slowly reduce stimulants such as caffeine, refined sugar, refined salt and so on. Enjoy some of the alkalizing juice on page 188 and any of the recipes from the Breakfast and Dinner chapters (see pages 100 and 148). On day 1, start your day with a bowl of Alchemical Oat Porridge (see page 104) during winter › spring; with Summertime Mineral-boosting Yogurt (see page 102) in spring › summer › autumn; or stewed apples (see page 109) in autumn › winter. Then have a bowl of Cleansing Kitchari (see page 157) for lunch and dinner. Repeat on days 2 and 3. Then for the next three days slowly reintroduce other foods. Start having some of the alkalizing juice again. Throughout the reset period you can also enjoy some of the Digestion-soothing Infusion on page 180 and plain hot water to drink. During the three days, rest and detox from screens as much as you can, and give yourself a gentle massage daily using the Nourishing Ghee Body Oil on page 81. You can burn some essential oils in the room as you do this (see page 33).

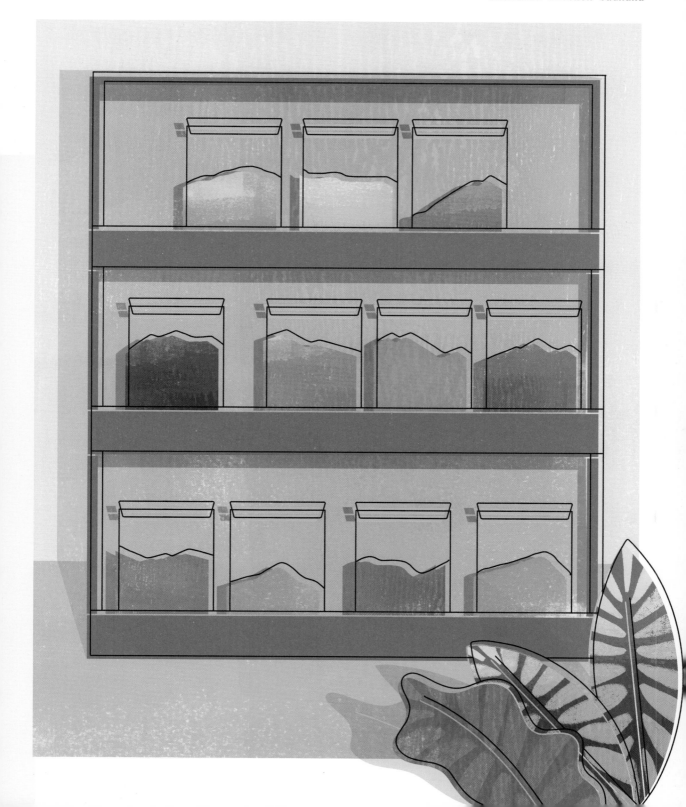

Spring

As the days become longer and the green shoots begin to appear, motivation often returns. I love to harness the renewed spring in my step and remove any sluggishness or excess heaviness that has accumulated over the winter.

In the kitchen

There is nothing lovelier than a spring clean. Cleaning the windows to let in returned light can be symbolic. Try using the Glass-cleaning Spray on page 33. I also find there is easy motivation this time of year to go through the kitchen cupboards and have a good rearrange, sort and clean. This sets up the kitchen for the season ahead.

Food

You may find you are more prone to coughs and colds or seasonal allergies as the body reacts to climatic changes. This is a great time for a bit of internal spring cleaning. Drink Nettle Leaf and Green Tea (see page 183), eat Savoury Oat Porridge for breakfast (see page 105), Cleansing Kitchari for lunch or dinner (see page 157), and for something sweet, try Anti-congestion Spicy Crackers (see page 166). Include seasonal greens such as dandelion shoots – these gently bitter leaves are awesome for the liver. This tea and food combination stimulates the digestive system and gently removes any stagnant *ama* (metabolic waste, see page 20).

Breathwork and movement

Now is a good time to get back outside, either speed walking, jogging or cycling at least three times per week. In my yoga practice and teaching I love to harness the spring energy and express a more dynamic style. When practising your breathwork as described on page 44, you may decide to do it with a little more vigour and bring in some arm movements. Try the following exercise sequence.

Chest and ribcage opener

1. Stand with feet hip-width apart. Raise your arms out to the sides until outstretched at chest height. Twist the upper torso from left to right, keeping your arms and head aligned with it and so moving along with it. Continue for 30 seconds. As you move, imagine you are clearing the space around you.

2. Place your hands on top of your shoulders. Bring the tips of your elbows towards each other in front of you. Then draw large circles with the elbows, bringing them up towards the ceiling, out to the sides, down underneath your chest and back towards each other. Repeat 5 times.

3. Finally interlace the fingers, turn the palms outward and raise them up towards the ceiling, outstretching the arms. Keeping your arms stretched up, bring your shoulders down and outwards, away from your ears. Take a few conscious breaths in this position. Then inhale and, as you exhale, gently lean over towards the right; inhale and return to the centre; then exhale and gently over towards the left; now inhale and return to centre. If it feels good, repeat a few more times.

Seasonal spice mixes

Each of the following herb-and-spice blends are ideal for a specific season and can be added to your cooking throughout that season.

Spring spice mix

During the spring we are looking to dry and clear out excess mucus or *kapha* we have accumulated over the winter. This spice mix can help. Black pepper is both heating and drying, and has specific properties related to the *pranavaha* channels (respiratory tract). Salt breaks down mucus. Rosemary is antimicrobial and supports the digestive system too, through its pungent and bitter tastes. Turmeric is bitter and pungent, acts as an expectorant and helps to clear *ama* (metabolic waste). As we clear the outside ground to prepare it for sowing seeds in late spring, so we can clear our internal ground too. Use ½ teaspoon per 4 servings, or to taste.

Makes 8 teaspoons

2 teaspoons black peppercorns
1 teaspoon turmeric
2 tablespoons finely chopped dried rosemary
1 teaspoon unrefined salt

Method

Grind the ingredients using a pestle and mortar. Store in an airtight container.

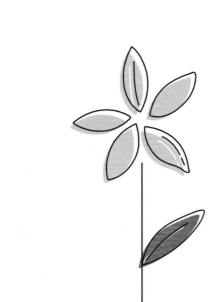

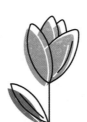
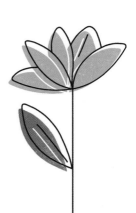

Summer

The warmth of the summer and length of the days can have a big impact on the kitchen environment. Food kept on the counter spoils more easily, but ferments take much less time to mature, owing to the higher temperature. We benefit from this heat too, with the digestive system working optimally and requiring less stimulation. In the summer, we require fewer calories, as we do not need as much fuel to stay warm. This lightens the load for the digestive system.

In the kitchen

If you have space to grow some outdoor herbs or other plants like beans, now is the perfect time to harness the drying heat of the summer. For example, mint that grows in abundance can be gathered and hung to dry. Beans that are harvested and dried now can then be saved for later in the year for soaking and cooking.

Food

As the heat of the summer begins to increase it is time to enjoy foods with cooling properties to prevent the bodily accumulation of too much heat. Luckily, nature gives us the perfect ingredients for this. Try the Cooling Cucumber and Celery Juice on page 184 or the Warm-weather Three-minute Couscous on page 142.

Breathwork and movement

The summer gifts us long days, so we can enjoy the coolness of the mornings and evenings outside. You can safely expose your skin to the sun at these times of day to top up your vitamin D stores. Due to the warm days the body is more relaxed, so we can benefit more readily from exercising outside. Seek out outdoor swimming possibilities. Swimming is a great exercise for the cardiovascular system, is easy on joints, regulates the breath and cools the body temperature in the heat. Try the following exercises to harness the summer energy, then collect yourself as the summer sun energizes you.

1. **Kneeling sun salute** Come to 'standing' on your knees. Place the palms of your hands together in front of your chest in prayer position and take a couple of conscious breaths here. Then, as you inhale, slowly bring your hands up overhead and then move them apart and outwards turning the palms up to the ceiling as you gaze upwards and lift your chest. Now, as you exhale, slowly bring your palms together above your head, move them down to your heart, turn them to face down toward the floor, then bend forward, place your palms on the floor and bring the forehead towards the floor. Inhale, come back up and travel

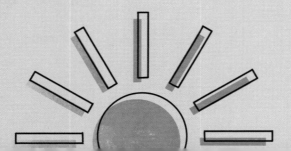

the hands all the way up to reach towards the sky again, then exhale and come down to the earth again as you did on the last exhalation. Repeat 5–10 times moving consciously and slowly, in sync with your breath, feeling the connection between the earth and sky.

2. ***Sitali pranayama*** This is excellent if you are feeling overheated or are suffering with menopausal hot flushes. It quickly cools you down: sit upright in a good posture. Stick out your tongue slightly and curl it if you can (this is genetic, so not everyone can). Alternatively make a tight 'O' shape with your mouth as if you are sucking through a straw. Inhale through the curled tongue or mouth, long slow and deep and exhale through your nose. Feel your body softening on the exhalation. Continue for up to one minute or until you feel cool.

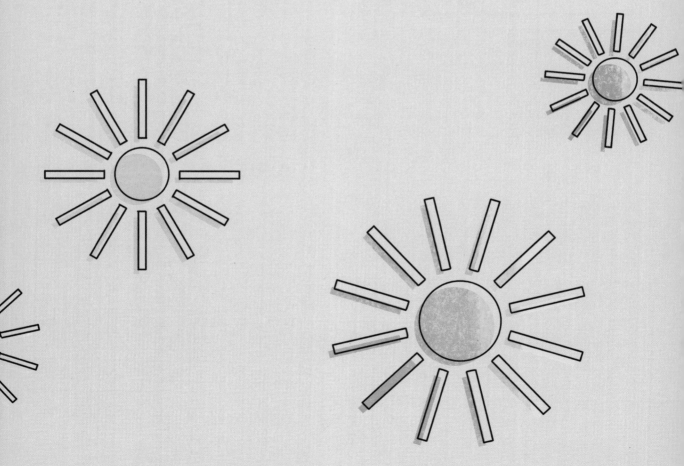

Summer spice mix

The summer sun can become quite intense and may cause us to accumulate excess heat in the body. In the kitchen we want to be using spices that are aromatic, have some sweet tastes and are not too heating. In this summer spice blend, coriander seeds support the urinary tract and help to cool any excess *pitta* (heat qualities, see page 14). Combining coriander with fennel and cumin further enhances this cooling quality, acting as an antidote to foods that would normally be heat promoting, such as tomatoes and chillies, which are common at the end of the summer. Adding coriander leaves further enhances the cooling aspect of this blend, as the leaves are more cooling than the seeds. Add ½–1 teaspoon spice mix per 4 servings.

Makes 8 teaspoons

6 teaspoons coriander seeds
2 teaspoons fennel seeds
2 teaspoons cumin seeds
2 tablespoons dried coriander leaves

Method
Grind the ingredients using a pestle and mortar. Store in an airtight container.

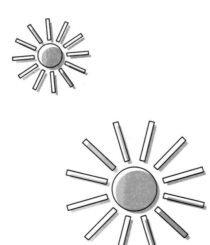

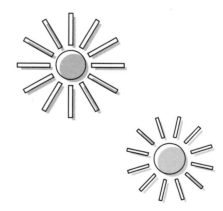

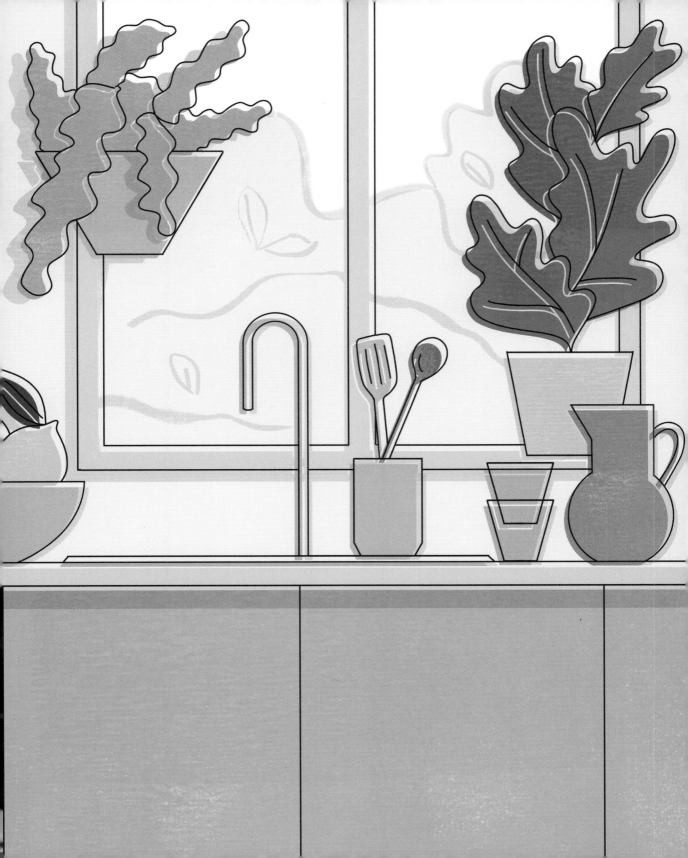

Autumn

Abundance is the key word for autumn. It is a very busy time of year in the kitchen as you maximize the benefits of the fruits of your labours, and those of others. There is so much free food available at this time of year, so it is great to get outside with friends and family in the last of the long days and hunt for blackberries, nuts and other treasures.

In the kitchen

The kitchen can be a hive of activity now as you prepare jams, such as Spiced Pumpkin Jam (see page 197), or ferments, such as Ginger, Red Cabbage and Beetroot Sauerkraut (see page 194). Ensure your cupboards are stocked with empty jam jars, wax discs and paper bags.

Food

You may find that your body is particularly dry at this time of year. It is the season of drying out – all the leaves are crisping up and falling. The drying heat of the summer is also likely to have left you feeling a little dry. From an Ayurvedic perspective this can affect the colon. The best way to deal with this is to drink some cleansing juices. The juice from local apples is perfect for this, as it can be mildly laxative and also has all the microbiota necessary to prepare the gut ahead of winter. In addition to this, add a little extra olive oil or ghee to your cooking to compensate for any dryness. Try adding a little more to the Nourishing Spiced Pumpkin Soup on page 150.

Breathwork and movement

As in the summer, it is still good to get outside and soak up the last rays of the sun before winter sets in. As the sun is less intense now, you can enjoy being outside more towards the middle of the day. If you have a garden or allotment, spending a lot of time preparing the garden ahead of the winter is great. Gardening is good for the mind, body and spirit. If you do not have a garden, head to the nearest woods or forest and enjoy the last moments of the leaves being on the trees, filling your lungs with freshly released oxygen from the trees and feeding the trees back with your freshly released carbon dioxide. You could try these exercises too, to steady yourself as the autumnal winds whip up around you.

1. **Tree pose** Stand near a wall or a tree if you need support. Stand with your feet hip-width apart. Feel the connection between your feet and the ground. Feel the counterforce of gravity lifting you up as your feet root into the ground. Feel some strength growing through your legs. Transfer your weight to your left foot and begin to bring the right foot off the ground, perhaps positioning it on the ankle of the left foot, perhaps on the calf or inner thigh (never on the knee). Then bring your palms together at your heart centre and allow the breath to flow. See how still you can become and feel the connection between your foot and the ground, and between your hands

pressed into each other. Trees move all the time, so do not worry about how much you are moving. Let the breath flow in and out 4–5 times, then bring the right foot down to the floor on an exhalation and change legs. Ensure you take time to root through the foot.

2. **Alternate nostril breathing** Sit upright with a good posture. Fold the index and middle fingers of your right hand down into your right palm. Raise the hand to your face and use your right thumb to close off your right nostril, take a lovely slow breath in through your left nostril, close off your left nostril with your ring finger and little finger, release your right thumb and let the breath roll out of your right nostril. Then breath in through your right nostril, close off the right nostril with your thumb, release your ring finger and little finger and exhale through your left nostril. Repeat this cycle 5–10 times, then relax your hand, allowing it to rest in your lap, and take 5 gentle, full breaths int hrough both of your nostrils.

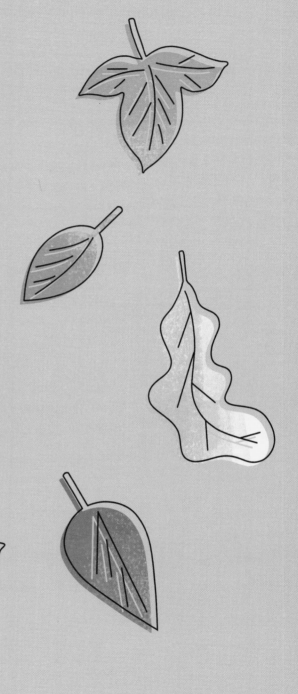

Autumn spice mix

During Autumn, the drying, cooling *vata*-type winds tend to increase. We need herbs that counteract this effect, as well as herbs that have antimicrobial properties, to prepare the body ahead of the winter. All the spices in this blend are gently warming, support lung health and are good for counterbalancing *vata*. Use ½–1 teaspoon spice blend per 4 servings.

Makes 10 teaspoons

2 tablespoons finely chopped dried sage leaves
2 teaspoon ground ginger
2 teaspoon dried thyme leaves
2 teaspoon ground cinnamon

Method

Grind the ingredients using a pestle and mortar. Store in an airtight container.

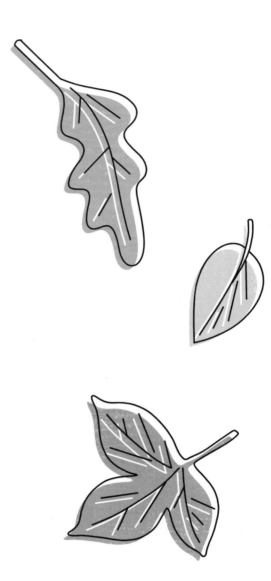

Winter

Batten down the hatches, light the candles and embrace the concept of *hygge*. Winter is the time to sit back and enjoy the fruits of your labour earlier in the year. It is a great time to self-nourish, plan for the year ahead and relax by the fire or radiator. Winter is often viewed negatively, owing to the lack of light and vitamin D creation, but it can instead be seen as a very romantic and magical time of year, during which we enjoy the preciousness of twinkling lights and warming aromatic smells coming from the kitchen.

In the kitchen

The kitchen really sings in the winter: the tantalizing smells of slow-cooked meals, soups and stews and aromatic drinks fill the air, making the taste buds tingle. Owing to the darkness outside you have more time to spend in the kitchen preparing meals that take longer to cook than in the summer. Recipes like comforting Slow-cooked Barley and Mung Beans (see page 154) or warming Mini-panforte (see page 168) are ideal for winter. Put on some heart-lifting music, light candles and invite friends or family over to bring your kitchen to life.

Food

In the winter we naturally need more calories in order to stay warm, so the food we eat tends to become richer and denser. We can also increase this warmth by adding warming aromatic spices, which has the additional benefit of helping us to digest the food and prevent the accumulation of unrequired *ama* (metabolic waste). It is really important to start the day with something warm, such as the Alchemical Oat Porridge on page 104.

Breathwork and movement

Attending local classes can be a supportive activity this time of year. The community feeling of being with other people is heartening on an emotional level. There are other advantages too. Feeling motivated to move might not come so easily during the winter months, and in a class setting you may find an increased desire for movement. You are also protected from the harsher elements outside. When time allows though, it is still good to wrap up in layers and get out into the midday elements and admire the sparse beauty of winter. Use the following exercises too, to keep yourself open and clear.

1. **Cat/Cow** Come onto your hands and knees. Inhale and move your sitting bones, chest and chin towards the ceiling into cow pose, then exhale and very slowly round the spine over to its comfortable maximum and release the head, looking downwards as you move into cat pose. Inhale and return to cow pose. Exhale, round the spine over and return to cat pose. Continue this slow flow 5–10 times, easing out the spine.

2. **Seated twist** Sit either upright on a chair and cross the left leg over the right leg, or cross legged and upright on the floor. Then turn towards your right, twisting the upper torso and opening up your chest, creating a gentle twist in the back. Support yourself with your right hand on the chair or floor behind you, and your left hand resting on your right knee. Hold the position and take a long gentle breath in through the nose, picture it

travelling down the spinal column, nourishing your cells as it goes, and then exhale the breath back up through the spinal column and out of the nose. Repeat 5–10 times, then unravel and repeat on the opposite side.

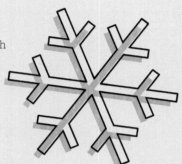

3. **Immunity stance** Come to standing with your feet hip-width apart. Raise both arms straight out to the side and elevate them to 30 degrees above shoulder height. Fold your fingers into the pads of your palms and leave your thumbs outstretched. Keep the top of your shoulders and neck relaxed. Take 5 deep conscious breaths in and out through your nose. Feel your arms extending out from the centre of your chest. Smile as you do this and feel bright and radiant.

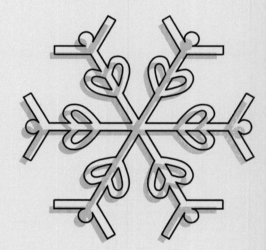

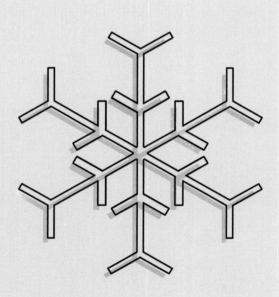

Winter spice mix

During the winter, we need three qualities in our food, which the spices in this blend provide. We need extra heat, in order to give an internal feeling of warmth to counterbalance the external coldness. We also need to help to promote the *agni* (digestive fire) – this must be strong to deal with the additional calories being consumed daily to keep us warm. Also, there is a tendency to accumulate excess mucus or *kapha* in the winter, so we need to support the lungs. All the spices in this blend are heating, antimicrobial, anti-inflammatory and break down mucus, so this is the ideal spice blend for winter. Use ½–1 teaspoon spice blend per 4 servings.

Makes 12 teaspoons

2 teaspoons garlic powder
4 teaspoons dried basil
2 teaspoons unrefined salt
2 teaspoons black peppercorns
2 teaspoons ground ginger

Method

Grind the ingredients using a pestle and mortar. Store in an airtight container.

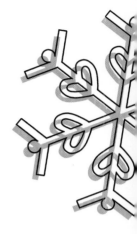

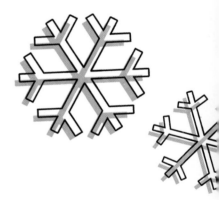

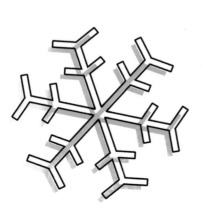

Nurturing edible plants _____

When you grow your own food, you have instant access to high-quality, ultra-fresh seasonal produce and, at the same time, you cut your carbon footprint and packaging waste. And as you slow down and connect to nature, you reap mental-health benefits too.

Whether we cultivate in gardens or allotments, patios or windowsills, we can have a positive impact on the environment. Growing produce allows us to take responsibility for maintaining good soil structure, and by planting a mixed range of crops, we encourage an abundance of wildlife. Local Permaculture courses can provide a wealth of knowledge about how to follow this way of life.

Indoor growing

Plants bring nature into your home and enliven a kitchen. Consider growing pot plants on windowsills or cultivating a living wall of herbs, such as basil, spinach and salad leaves. You can dedicate different areas of your kitchen to varying lifecycles of herbs.

Kitchens tend to remain at a fairly constant temperature all year round, so in temperate climates they provide ideal environments for cultivating herbs suited to growing outside only in the summer months. Given the right treatment, oregano, sweet marjoram, chives, basil and sage can thrive in an indoor environment. Also, try growing wheatgrass or microleaf mixed salads, which grow well indoors and are packed with nutrients.

Patio growing

If you have a patio, growing seasonal herbs, such as sage, thyme, parsley, mint, dill and French tarragon, gives you access to a huge range of flavours. Also try salads, sorrel leaves and vegetables such as tomatoes, cucumbers and courgettes.

Garden or allotment

Given enough space, you can grow a good variety of vegetables in every season. I am a huge fan of 'no-dig' gardening, which tends to take any stress out of gardening to give you maximum enjoyment. Let nature do the work for you, especially if you are time-poor. Then, simply plant the things you love to eat and that are suited to the environment in which you live.

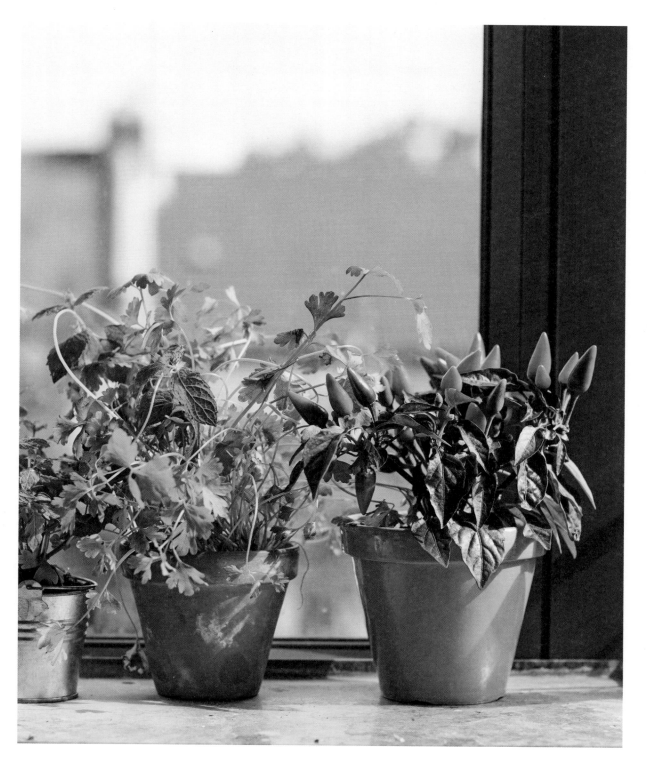

Sprouting and fermenting

These living organic processes bring *Prana* (life force) into your kitchen and give you a deep connection with nature all year round. Watching the daily progress of a seed sprouting is watching life itself in action.

Sprouting

Sprouting specially purchased non-GMO beans and seeds can be a hugely satisfying process, and one that provides you with wonderful nutrition. Sprouted seeds and beans are full of metabolic potential. As their energy is unleashed through the germination process, they release many of the stored vitamins and minerals that are locked into unsprouted seeds by phytic acid, which are then more bioavailable to us. Research shows that sprouting increases the amount of protein available per seed or bean, while reducing anti-nutritional factors such as lectins and oxalates, which can adversely affect the digestibility of the protein.

It is really important when sprouting that you follow excellent, even ramped up, hygiene practices to prevent the growth of harmful bacteria. Any jars or kit you are using must be sterilized and all kitchen surfaces must be super clean.

If you have success growing herbs from seed, you will be able to sprout – in fact, it is easier. You do not need any soil and the living plants are ready to eat after 2–4 days. There are many different types of sprouting equipment available, but all you really need is an upturned jam jar with a lid full of small holes and something to prop it up with. Try making one yourself using a jam jar and a square of muslin (see below) or buy a sprouting starter kit.

My favourite bean to sprout is the mung bean, because it only takes a couple of days and it is easy to digest. I also like to sprout chickpeas, as it halves their cooking time (see my recipe for Sprouted Chickpea Hummus on page 200).

Look out for organic and non-GMO seeds and beans that are intended for sprouting, certified organic and from the nearest geographical region.

Place 40g (1½oz) or your desired amount of mung bean seeds in a sterilized jam jar (see page 196 for sterilizing instructions). Add enough filtered water to cover the beans by 5cm (2in). Cover the mouth of the jar with some muslin (cheesecloth) and secure with an elastic band. Leave to soak overnight.

The next morning, drain the water out of the beans. Pour in some fresh filtered water, swill it around in the jar, then turn the jar upside down and allow the water to pour out into the sink through the muslin. Now balance the upturned jar in the bowl, leaning it up against the edge of the bowl. This will allow air to flow around the mouth of the jar and catch any draining liquid. Position the bowl in a dark corner of the kitchen, out of direct sunlight.

Around 5 hours later, repeat the rinsing and draining process. This act of caring for these magical sprouts is like a moving meditation. Repeat again later in the day, and 3 times over the next day. By now some tails should have appeared on the mung beans. You can allow them to sprout further, and when they have sprouted to your desired amount, use them. Add to the compost pile anything looking a bit furry, or that looks or smells mouldy.

Finally, thoroughly cook your sprouts at above 65°C (150°F) to ensure great digestion and safety.

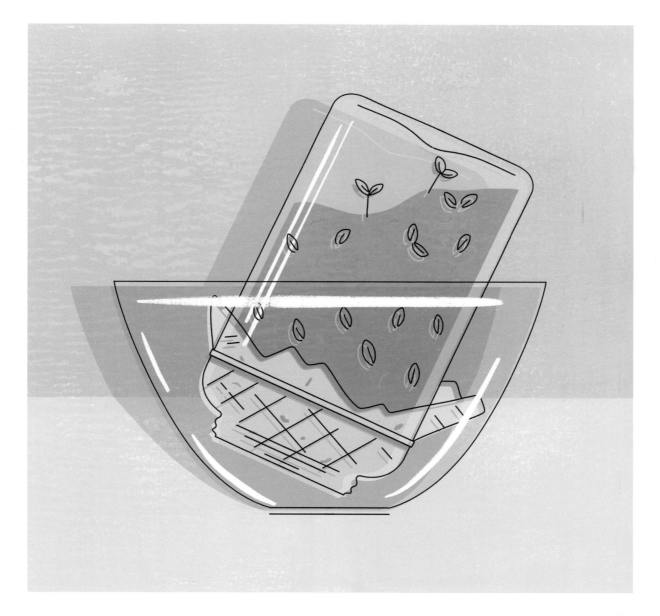

Fermenting

The skill of fermentation has been around for millennia and is well documented in Ayurveda (see the recipe for Ginger, Red Cabbage and Beetroot Sauerkraut on page 194 as an example). It is a true gift from nature – as with sprouting, you gain through nature's input and end up with something that is metabolically richer or, at the very least, interestingly different to what you started with. Friendly bacteria step in to give birth to whole new types of foods that have wonderful benefits for our *agni* (digestive fire).

The process also offers a great way of preventing food waste. It enables you to prolong the lifespan of produce and, therefore, save it for the future – which means you prevent the need to expend as many food miles in times of less natural abundance, such as during the depths of winter.

Once you begin fermenting, suddenly you see food preservation opportunities everywhere. The only limitation is the amount of preserving jars you have available! When selecting ingredients to ferment, it is a question of finding what is palatable to you and what makes you feel good. Any vegetables or fruits that are about to begin spoiling can be turned into a form of sauerkraut, pickle, relish or a drink. Dairy produce that is approaching its end can be turned into hundreds of different delectable foods, such as Cumin Labneh (see page 201). Grains can also be fermented.

Very strong acidic ferments can be too intense for some already fiery digestive systems, in which case, simply reduce the fermentation time to make a lighter one. This is the beauty with making your own products – you can leave them for as many or as few days as you wish.

As with sprouting, excellent kitchen hygiene is a must when fermenting, and if mould is appearing below the ferment line, or if the ferment does not look right, then you should allow that product's life to continue in the compost bin instead.

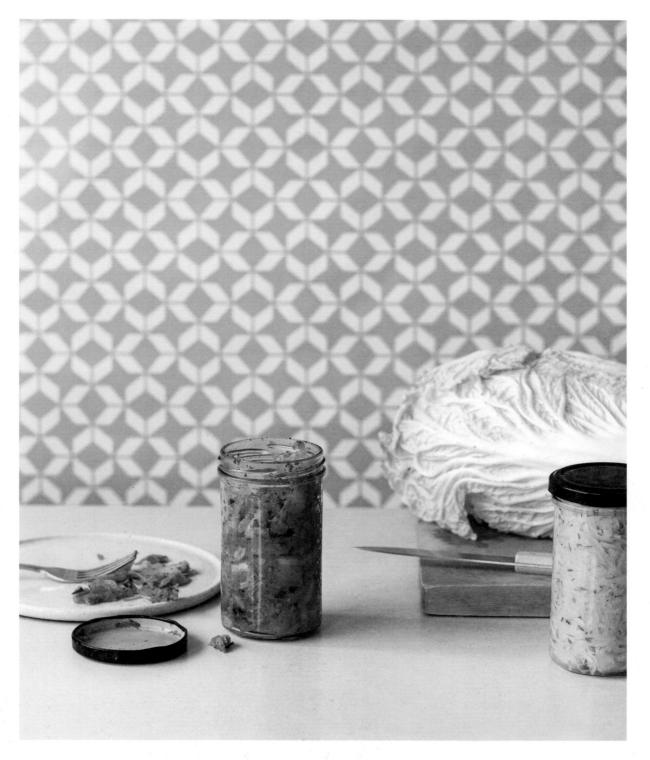

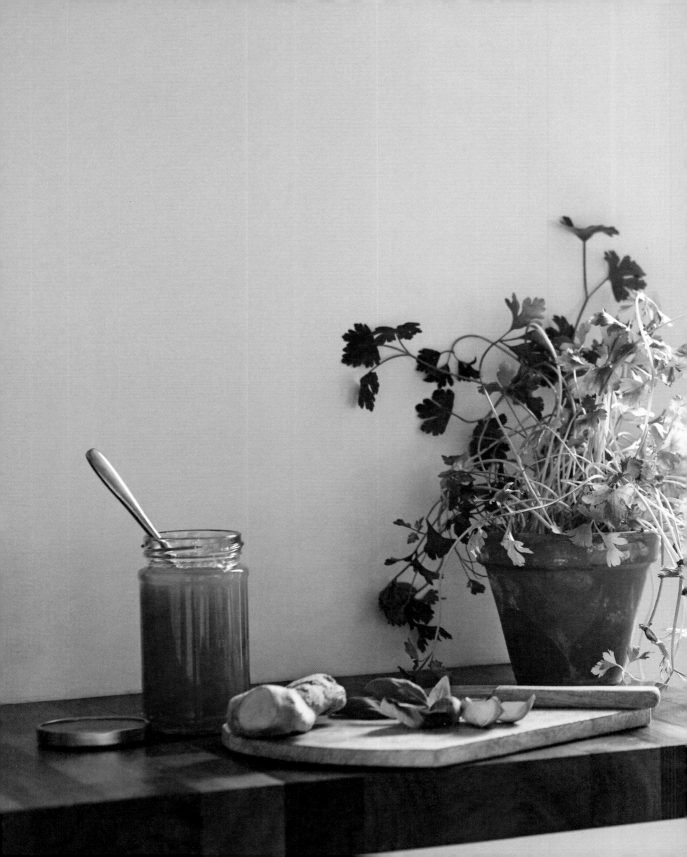

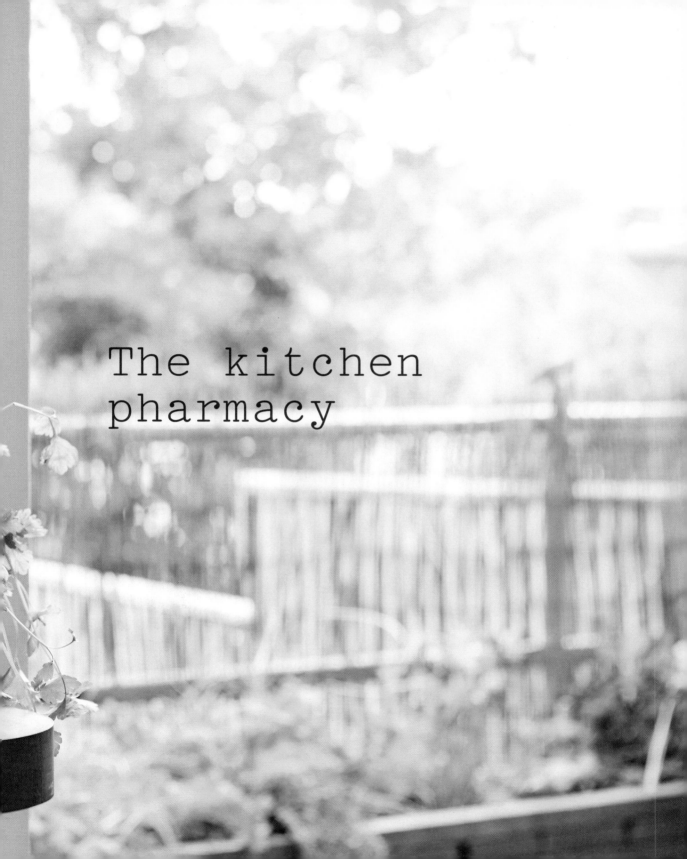

The kitchen pharmacy

Simple kitchen remedies _____

In Ayurveda it is understood that there is nothing in this universe that cannot be made into a medicine. As the kitchen is where we create things to ingest, in addition to food and drinks we can also make simple remedies.

The special properties, qualities and medicinal uses of all plants, animals, milks, fats, minerals, metals and even types of water are listed in Ayurveda. If you were to visit an Ayurvedic pharmacy you would see that it is like a large industrial kitchen, with an oversized herb garden attached. The fragrance inside, coming from huge vats of bubbling oils, is entrancing. People sit meditatively, grinding herbs with pestle and mortar or rolling pills by hand. A single preparation can take days or weeks to make.

Much of this knowledge has spilled into people's homes. Indians regularly use herbs and spices to make remedies for minor ailments in their own kitchens. This is a way of life as opposed to an extra-special thing they do.

Key Ayurvedic ingredients

Over the years I have instructed people on how to make tonics and remedies out of ingredients they can readily find in their own kitchens, or using special herbs I recommend. In order to keep food miles down and local beneficial properties high, opposite I provide an Ayurvedic take on mostly locally grown herbs and foods that you can incorporate into your own kitchen pharmacy, outlining the qualities and properties of each ingredient.

Remedies for common ailments

For minor ailments, your Ayurveda Kitchen can be your first port of call when it comes to remedies. The following preparations are all simple to make.

Basil

Basil is the most glorious plant to have on a kitchen windowsill. It loves the warmth and will thrive there all year-round, although you may need to keep growing new plants if you use it a lot. With different variations of the genus all over the world, it truly is a global plant. In India it is known as holy basil or *tulsi* and is regarded as a highly auspicious plant that is full of *sattva* (complete harmony).

One of the best uses of basil, from a kitchen-pharmacy perspective, is in treating colds or the accumulation of mucus. It is a brilliant herb to use during the transition from winter into spring when there is a lot of excess dampness.

Action Heating.

Tastes Pungent and bitter.

Medicinal properties Antibacterial, antiseptic, carminative, decongestant, diaphoretic and antispasmodic.

Internal use Basil Infusion (see page 77) is great in cases of fever and coughs and colds where mucus is a dominant feature. It can also help with sore throats.

External use I have used the juice of the leaves and the leaves themselves successfully to treat fungal toenail infections and other fungal skin diseases. Squeeze the juice from several leaves onto the affected nail, then place the squeezed leaves onto the toenail, secure with a sock or micropore tape and leave until the next application the following day, unless the plaster falls off before. Repeat daily for two weeks.

In cooking The wonderful properties of basil will be imparted to the dish, although in a more diluted form than they would be in a medicinal application.

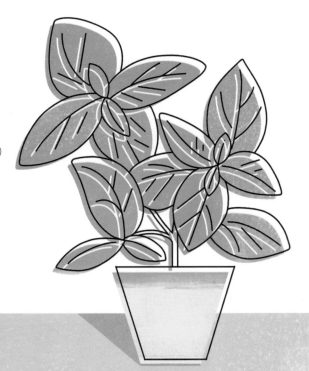

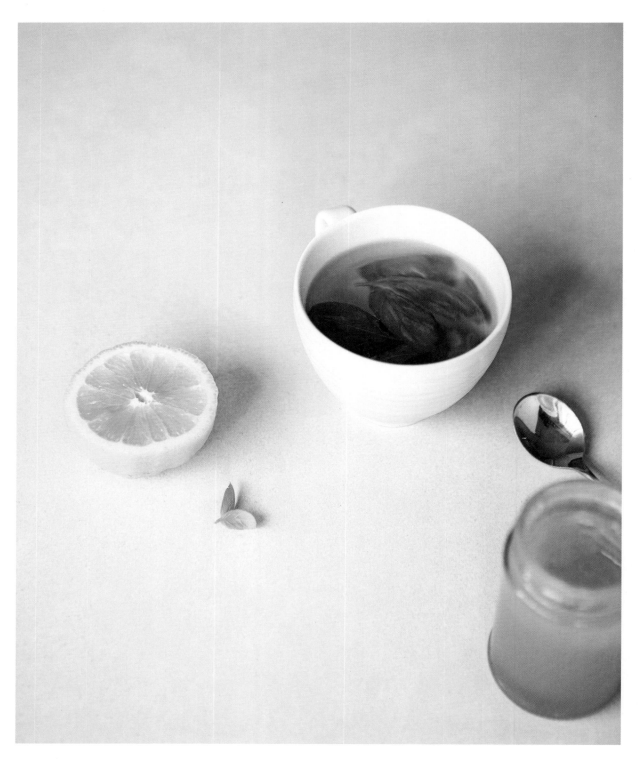

Basil Infusion

Make this tea if you feel you are suffering
from a fever, cough or cold-type virus. You
can make 2–3 cups of this across the day.
In Ayurveda we use a type of basil known
as *tulsi*, which has strong anti-viral and
anti-bacterial properties. I have successfully
grown it from seed on my sunny windowsill.

Makes 1 dose

small handful of fresh basil leaves
1 mug water at 60°C (140°F)
2 tablespoons lemon juice
1 teaspoon local unprocessed honey

Put the basil leaves into the mug of hot water
and leave to infuse for 5 minutes. Stir in the
lemon juice and, just before serving, the honey.

Coriander

Coriander can be tricky to grow year-round. There is a type of Vietnamese coriander that often grows better indoors and may be picked multiple times yet continues to grow. Coriander is suitable for treating all types of imbalance and is particularly useful when you need a cooling herb for irritation. Both the leaves and seeds can be used.

Action Seeds are heating, leaves are cooling.

Tastes Bitter, sweet and astringent.

Medicinal properties Antihistamine-like action, anti-inflammatory, carminative, diuretic, diaphoretic.

Internal use Coriander leaves can help to ease an inflamed sore throat. Both leaves and seeds have a special affinity with the urinary system, so are helpful in treating cystitis, as they have a mild diuretic property. The fresh juice of the leaves is particularly beneficial for allergies and hay fever when you want an antihistamine-type effect. An infusion (see opposite) or decoction of the seeds can be useful when there is excess acidity or inflammation within the digestive system.

External use The juice or crushed leaves can be applied to red, itchy skin rashes. Press a small bundle of the leaves onto a teaspoon to extract the juice. Gently apply the juice to the irritated area, then put the mashed leaves on top. Leave for approximately 10 minutes. Use this remedy as often as it gives you relief.

In cooking Coriander helps to cool and balance out spicy dishes, especially those containing chilli, peppers and tomatoes.

Coriander Infusion

This tea is good for your digestive system if you are prone to acidity and inflammation. It is also supportive for the urinary system and acts as a mild diuretic. Have a cup after breakfast and another after lunch.

Makes 1 dose

¼ teaspoon coriander seeds
¼ teaspoon fennel seeds
200ml (⅓ pint) water at 80°C (175°F)

Place the whole seeds in a small tea pot and pour over the measured water. Leave to infuse for 5 minutes, then pour the tea through a tea strainer and serve immediately.

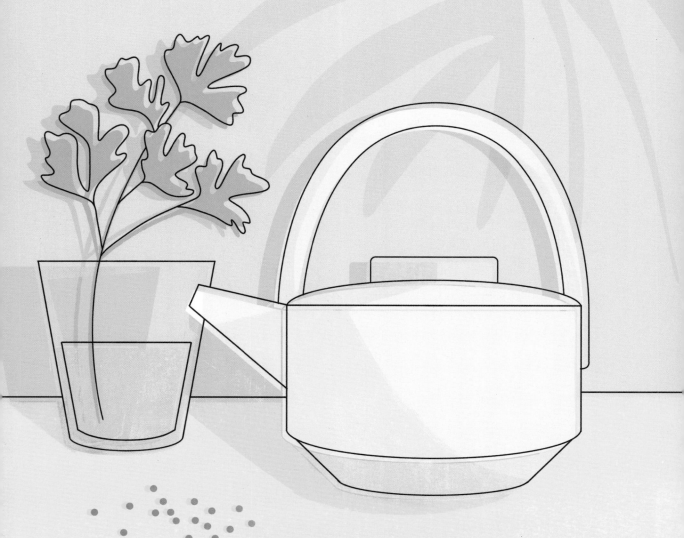

Ghee

Ghee (clarified butter) helps to soothe inflammation within the digestive system and promotes the building of good HDL cholesterol in the body – so long as it is used in moderation. It contains an ideal ratio of saturated and unsaturated fats, where the saturated fats are mostly short-chain fatty acids, which can be easily metabolized. It also contains butyric acid, a short-chain fatty acid that benefits the body in many ways, including boosting the immune system.

Action Cooling.

Taste Sweet.

Medicinal properties Anabolic, antacid, mild laxative, tonic, has rejuvenating properties and promotes vigour.

Internal use Ghee can be added to water, milk, porridge and other foods to take as a medicine to help calm excessive acidity. It can also be taken to help soften hard stools and give more lustre to the skin.

External use Ghee is fabulous for healing wounds and for moisturizing very dry chapped skin. Using a clean spoon to remove some ghee from your container, apply the ghee to rough skin on elbows, hands or on dry skin anywhere on the body. Reapply daily and watch your skin heal.

In cooking Ghee is readily available to buy and you will find a recipe for it on page 196. Also known as clarified butter, it can be used to cook with daily. In cooking, stick to 1–2 teaspoons per person across the course of one day. If you are suffering with very dry skin or excess acidity, add ½–1 teaspoon ghee to your porridge for breakfast.

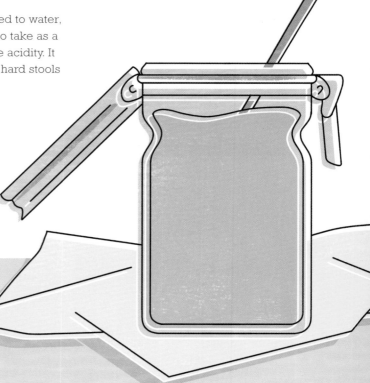

Nourishing Ghee Body Oil

This silky smooth oil works wonders for very dry skin. Before use, ensure you put the container on a radiator or immerse it in hot water for a few minutes to allow the ghee to melt and homogenize. Use an 80ml (2¾fl oz) glass storage bottle. The essential oil is an optional addition. Do use your favourite, but I generally recommend lavender. This product will keep in a cool, dark place for up to six months, but it is so lovely you will probably use it up within a couple of weeks!

A gentle daily massage using this body oil can be an enjoyable part of your Seasonal Reset Ritual (see page 52). In a warm bathroom, undress and sit on a towel. With a loving, gentle touch, take your time to slowly anoint your whole body with some warmed oil, working from your extremities towards your centre. Allow it to soak in for 5 minutes, then shower or immerse yourself in a bath.

Makes 75g (2¾oz)

60ml (4 tablespoons) olive oil
15g (½oz) ghee (see page 196)
few drops essential oil (optional)

Put the olive oil and ghee into a saucepan and gently warm to allow the ghee to liquefy. Take the pan off the heat, stir in the essential oil (if using), then pour the mixture into a glass bottle. Allow to cool completely before securing the lid.

Ginger

Ginger is known in Ayurveda as 'the universal or great medicine' and is probably my number-one go-to kitchen spice for digestive and respiratory ailments. It is the best medicine for all *vata* disorders (see page 17). It is super effective at bringing the digestive system back online, reduces swelling and it also has strong anti-inflammatory properties. However, ginger is heating, so in conditions where there are, say, ulcers, it should be used with caution. (You can grow stem ginger at home, but it is less pungent than regular root ginger, owing to the cooler climate. As an added bonus, however, you can use its leaves in cooking.)

In Ayurveda, fresh root ginger and dried powdered ginger are treated as two different medicines, with two different names, and have slightly different actions, as you will see below.

Action Fresh root ginger – heating and moistening; dry powdered root ginger – heating and drying.

Taste Pungent.

Medicinal properties Anti-inflammatory, analgesic, antiemetic, carminative, expectorant and stimulant.

Internal use Ginger is one of the best spices for improving the quality of digestion. You can use it to ease indigestion, nausea, vomiting, loss of appetite and abdominal pain, to name just a few of the digestive complaints it can help to heal. By improving the quality of *agni* (digestive fire), *ama* (metabolic waste) is reduced. Ginger is also known for its special action on the respiratory system and can be used to treat coughs and colds. Here, the difference between fresh and dry comes in to play. Dry ground ginger helps to dry the mucous linings within the respiratory tract, whereas fresh ginger liquifies mucus and helps to expectorate it. Ginger is very heating, so should be used in moderation in conditions where heat is a dominant feature, as well as in the summer.

External use A paste can be made out of ginger to apply to areas causing arthritis-type pain or joint pain. If there is swelling that is cold to the touch around joints, or prolonged stiffness, make a paste by mixing 1 teaspoon ground ginger with 1 teaspoon water and apply this to the affected area. Leave for 5–10 minutes, then wash off. Wash it off if, at any point, your skin feels a burning sensation. This preparation is unsuitable for those with sensitive skin.

In cooking Both dried and fresh ginger can be used widely in cooking. Ginger helps to improve the digestion of whatever food it is combined with, so add it to dishes containing foods you normally find harder to digest.

Ginger Decoction

This warming decoction is great for those moments when you feel as though you are coming down with a cough or cold. At these times, keep your diet light, prioritize your activities and rest as much as you can. Also do something that makes you smile. This boosts your neurotransmitters, which will in turn boost your immune system. Drink two small cups of the strained tea during the day.

Makes 2 doses

1cm (½in) piece of fresh root ginger
5 cloves
10 black peppercorns
3 cardamom pods, lightly crushed
5cm stick of cinnamon
1 litre (1¾ pints) water

Place all the ingredients in a saucepan and bring to a boil, then simmer until the liquid has reduced to one-third of its original quantity (approximately 375ml / 13fl oz). Serve half the decoction in a small mug immediately, and reserve a portion to reheat and serve later.

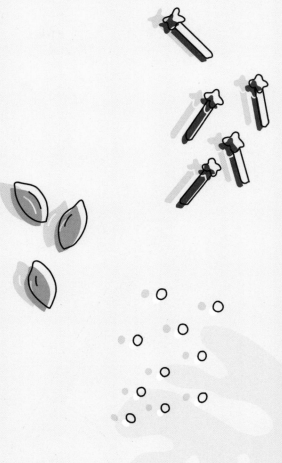

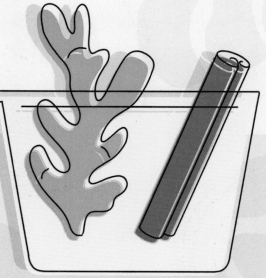

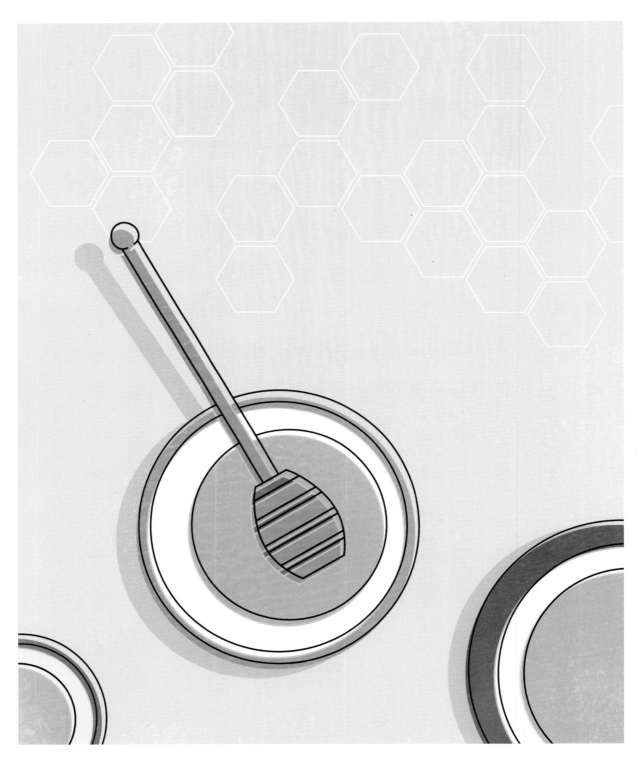

Honey

Honey is one of nature's wonders. It takes 12 bees to produce 1 teaspoon of honey. Ayurveda recommends you acquire raw (not heat-treated), local, unfiltered honey (which is unsuitable for children under 12 months).

Ayurveda differentiates between honey that is over or less than one year old. Old honey is considered to have a more drying effect on the body and has a special ability to reduce adipose/fat tissue. Freshly collected honey is considered to be much more nourishing. For those suffering from obesity or excess stubborn fat, try starting each day with a cup of warm water with 1 teaspoon honey stirred into it.

Honey has another special function. In Ayurveda, it is known as being *yogavahi*. It contains compounds that, when ingested, make it easier for the body to absorb the active ingredients in other medicinal foods. So it is a medicine in itself and an ideal carrier for other foods with medicinal properties, as it helps to unlock those properties for the body. Ghee has this same special characteristic, so you often see it being used as a carrier for other medicines.

Action Heating.

Tastes Sweet, astringent.

Medicinal Properties Antibacterial, antifungal, demulcent, expectorant, nutritive.

Internal use If you suffer from hay fever, as a preventative measure at the end of February/beginning of March, take 1 teaspoon honey from a local apiary in the morning. It is best to eat it straight from the spoon – and it's the most delicious way! Because it is full of pollen from local flowers, it is believed it can help the body to recognize these pollens as safe and not worthy of a hyper reaction, thus providing the body with local immune-supporting elements. In addition, honey has a 'scraping' effect and helps to clear mucus from the chest, which is a good thing to do ahead of hay-fever season. If you have excess mucus, a productive cough or laboured digestion, try the Honey and Trikatu Electuary on page 87.

External use Honey works wonders on mouth ulcers or minor abrasions. Simply apply a big dab to a mouth ulcer. Keep your mouth open and your tongue away from the area while it goes to work. When it becomes uncomfortable, you can close your mouth. Classically, we also use it on burns. There have been many global trials[4] demonstrating the effectiveness of honey for use in modern healthcare settings. It is used especially for treating superficial and partial-thickness burns and ulcers. Special manuka honey dressings are now regularly administered.

In cooking As honey is such a special product of nature, it is never cooked in Ayurveda. Cooking denatures the precious enzymes that are so good in it. It is also considered that cooking it turns honey into *ama*. So if you are making a jam like the Spiced Pumpkin Jam on page 197 with honey, or adding it to a warm drink like the Basil Infusion on page 77, wait for the drink to cool as much as possible before stirring in the honey directly before you begin to drink, at which point the drink will be not far off body temperature.

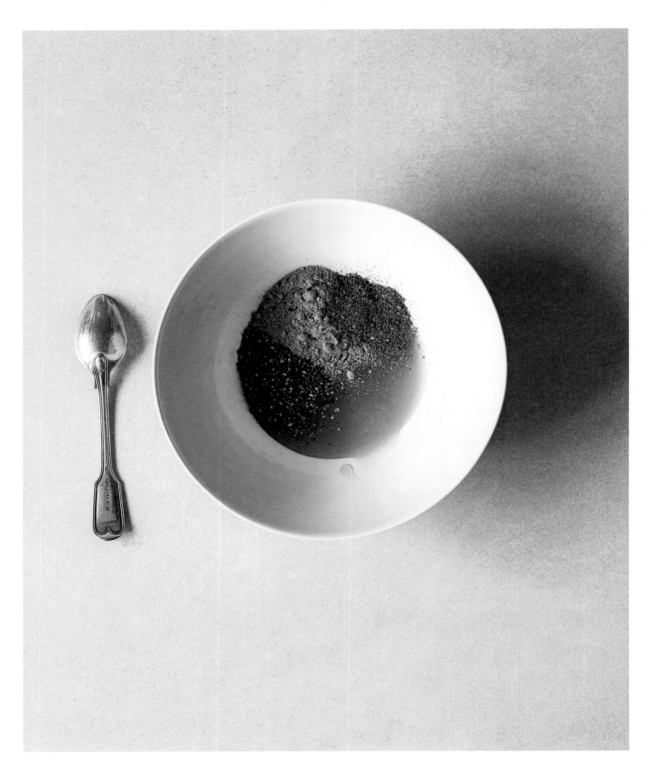

Honey and Trikatu Electuary

Warning – this treatment is very spicy to taste! If you are suffering from a wet cough, struggling to digest your meals or if you generally feel sluggish and heavy, try using this lickable paste. Dip the tip of a teaspoon into this mixture (you only need between ⅛–¼ teaspoon), lick the end of the spoon and feel the warmth wash over you. Everyone's perception of taste is slightly different, so some will find it more heating than others. Take it twice a day using a clean teaspoon to avoid contaminating the product. Do not use if you have gastritis or are suffering from any excessively heating or drying complaints, or if you are pregnant.

Tri means 'three' and *katu* means 'pungent'. Classically one of the three pungent spices it is made from is *pippali* (long pepper), but this can be hard to obtain. I have substituted with thyme, which has similar properties. Alternatively, you can buy Trikatu powder from reputable Ayurvedic suppliers. Trikatu boosts the natural production of hydrochloric acid (which the stomach needs for digestion) and supports the production of bile and digestive enzymes, thereby helping to clear *ama* (metabolic waste).

Makes 24 doses

1 teaspoon ground ginger
1 teaspoon ground black pepper
1 teaspoon ground dried thyme
 (or *pippali*, if you can find it)
6 teaspoons raw local honey

Simply mix all the ingredients together and store in a small, sterile airtight jar (see page 196 for sterilizing instructions) for up to three months.

Sage

Sage is one of the very few herbs that is available year-round in the northern hemisphere. It goes to sleep over winter, but its leaves are usually still available for picking. It becomes somewhat straggly towards the end of winter, when it prepares for the next year's growth. Sage is great for drying up excess mucus and secretions in the body, so is ideal for use throughout the winter into the spring, when coughs and colds can be more present.

Action Heating.

Tastes Pungent, bitter and astringent.

Medicinal properties Diaphoretic, expectorant and nervine.

Internal use Sage is well known for its ability to help with night sweats in menopausal women. Try infusing 4 sage leaves in a mug of water at 80°C (175°F) for 5 minutes and drink before bed. As mentioned above, it also helps to dry out colds and can be combined with honey and lemon.

External use Sage can be combined with other herbs and boiling water to create a wonderful airway-clearing Sage Steam treatment (see opposite).

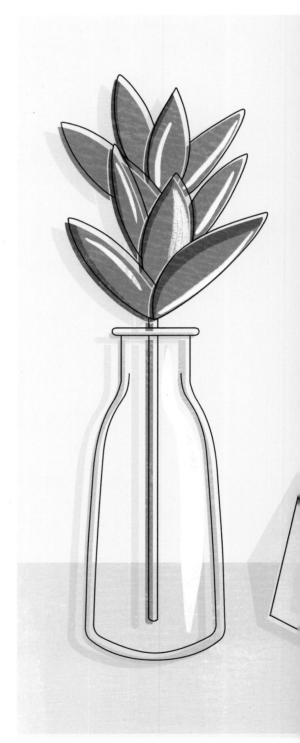

Sage Steam

Using steam inhalation with this blend
of herbs is useful when you have a cold or
congested chest. The plants used all have
antibacterial and congestion-relieving
properties that are released by the heat
of the water. Facial steaming is also great
for cleansing the skin.

For 1 steam session

1 litre (1¾ pints) boiling water
1 tablespoon sage leaves
1 tablespoon thyme leaves
1 tablespoon rosemary leaves

Pour the measured boiling water into a large,
wide-brimmed bowl. Add the leaves, then
cover the bowl with a bath towel and leave
to infuse for 3 minutes.

Lift up the towel on one side of the bowl
and pop your head underneath it, above the
steaming water, so you can inhale the steam.
Gather up the loose ends of towel around
you as much as possible, to trap the steam,
although you may need to retain a small
opening to allow enough steam to escape to
enable you to inhale. As your sinuses begin to
open, you may find you can start to inhale the
steam more easily through your nose, and
you can therefore gradually close up the
opening. Remain in position, inhaling the
steam, for 3–5 minutes, until you feel some
relief from your symptoms.

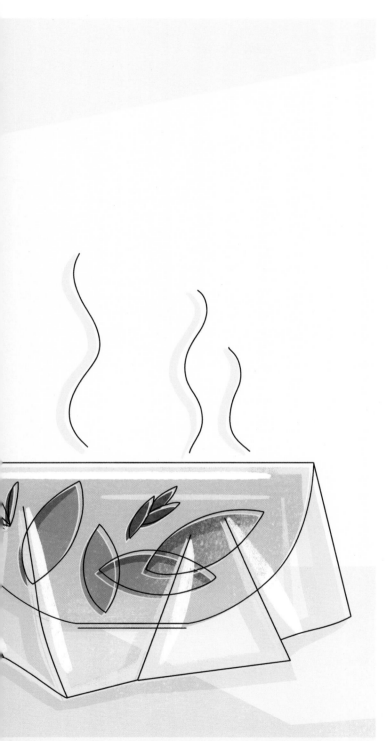

Salt

There are many types of salt, such as sea salt, rock salt, Himalayan salt and black salt, all with different properties. However, we do not need to get too picky, here – use any unrefined salt. Salt that has not been refined has a higher mineral profile, which is more useful for the body. Salt can be used medicinally to good effect at the right moment, as described below.

Action Heating.

Taste Salty.

Medicinal properties Anti-diuretic, breaks mucus, gentle laxative and promotes salivation.

Internal use Salt can be used in a mouth or throat gargle (see opposite). It helps to clear and prevent dental infection and treat sore throats, especially when combined with turmeric.

External use Bathing in a bath tub with a couple of tablespoons of unrefined salt can help to heal scratches, pimples and damaged skin, as well as restore the proper pH balance of the skin.

In cooking Ayurveda strongly recommends using unrefined salt, whether it be sea salt or rock salt. Unrefined salt contains many trace minerals that are important for health. In Ayurveda, we recommend the total daily unrefined salt intake for an average adult is around ½ teaspoon (4g). Too much salt puts pressure on the kidneys and causes a kind of dehydration that cannot be remedied by drinking water. Table salt (refined salt) often has iodine added to it to prevent goitre. Seaweed, which contains iodine, can be added to unrefined salt to similar effect.

Salt and Turmeric Throat Gargle

If you are suffering from a sore throat, swollen gums or dental problems, try this gargle, which can help to prevent and clear mild infections. Two or three times a day, pour a small amount into a glass and gargle and swish the liquid around your mouth for a few minutes before spitting it out. Repeat for a few days. If symptoms have not cleared by that point, seek help from a dentist or doctor.

Makes 2–3 doses

200ml ($\frac{1}{3}$ pint) water
small pinch of unrefined salt
small pinch of turmeric powder

Put the ingredients into a saucepan and simmer for 5 minutes. This is an essential step, as it activates the turmeric and infuses the properties of both the salt and turmeric into the water. Allow the mixture to cool, then transfer to a small jug, cover and keep on the countertop. Use at room temperature, on the day of making.

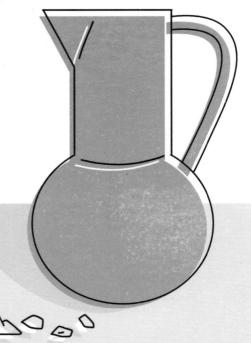

Mint

Mint grows prolifically outside in the summer months in the northern hemisphere and inside during the winter, and there are many different types, varying in pungency. If you do not plant it in a pot, you will quickly find it will have taken over an entire bed. It can easily and quickly be dried ahead of the winter, when its leaves will fall and the plant will become dormant until the spring.

Action Initially heating with a cooling feeling, then pungent after digestion.

Taste Pungent.

Medicinal properties Analgesic, antispasmodic, carminative, diaphoretic, refrigerant and stimulant.

Internal use Mint is wonderful for the digestive system. It is especially good as an appetizer, as it prepares the digestive system ahead of a meal – either chew a couple of leaves or prepare a tea by steeping some fresh leaves in ½ mug hot water for 5 minutes, and drinking around 15 minutes before your meal.

Mint can be a good alternative to ginger if you find ginger too heating. It can help with nervous agitation in the digestive system in particular, calming the condition prior to eating. Alternatively, if you have a good appetite, you can instead enjoy it as described above but after a meal, to give fresh breath and promote digestion of the meal.

External use Mint's special simultaneous heating and cooling properties make it helpful all year round. Extracting the juice from the leaves and mixing it with water creates an excellent mouth gargle.

In cooking Owing to its digestion-enhancing properties, mint is a great herb to use liberally in dishes.

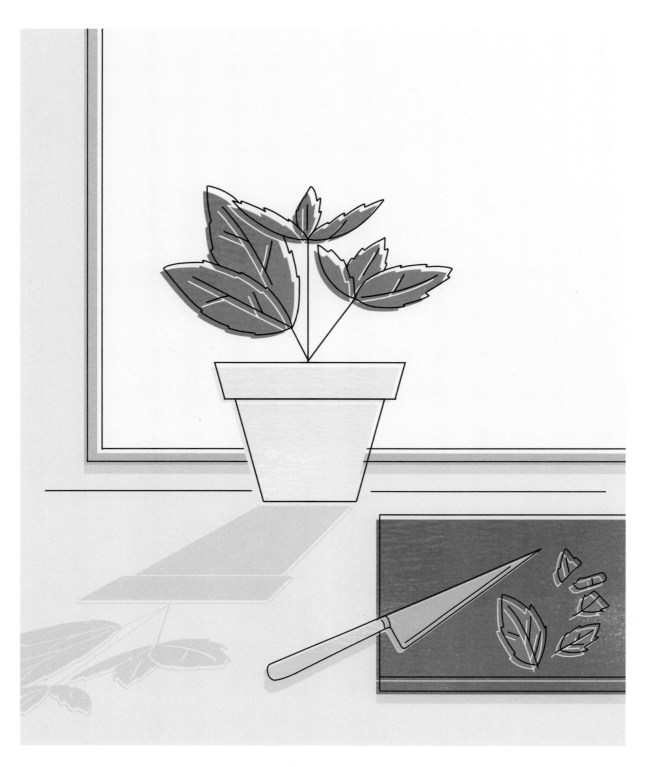

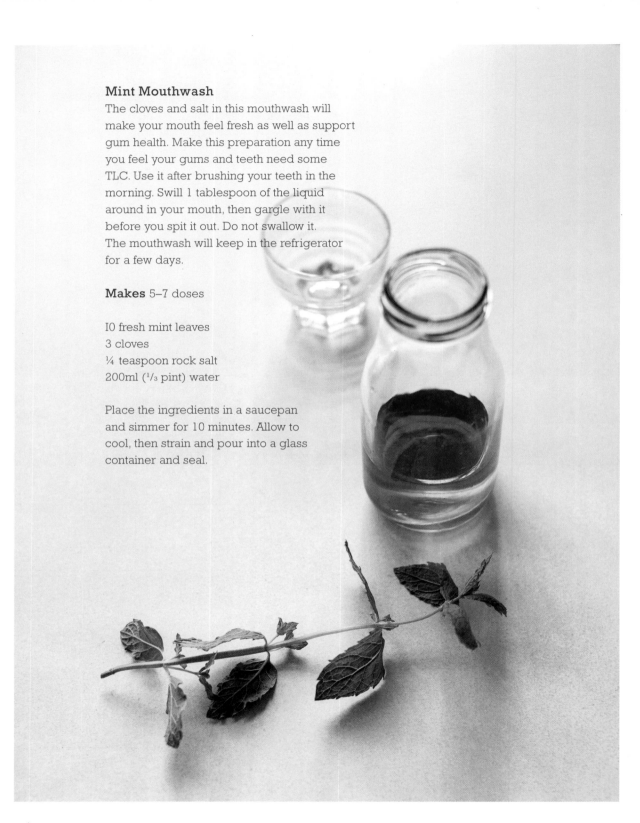

Mint Mouthwash

The cloves and salt in this mouthwash will make your mouth feel fresh as well as support gum health. Make this preparation any time you feel your gums and teeth need some TLC. Use it after brushing your teeth in the morning. Swill 1 tablespoon of the liquid around in your mouth, then gargle with it before you spit it out. Do not swallow it. The mouthwash will keep in the refrigerator for a few days.

Makes 5–7 doses

10 fresh mint leaves
3 cloves
¼ teaspoon rock salt
200ml (⅓ pint) water

Place the ingredients in a saucepan and simmer for 10 minutes. Allow to cool, then strain and pour into a glass container and seal.

Turmeric

Turmeric has received so much attention recently in wellbeing circles, owing to its incredible anti-inflammatory properties. It is often combined with ghee and black pepper to increase the bioavailability of these properties.

Action Heating, then pungent after digestion.

Tastes Bitter and astringent.

Medicinal properties Antibacterial, antifungal, antimicrobial, anti-inflammatory and clears mucus and *ama* (waste matter) toxins.

Internal use Consuming turmeric as a spice regularly can help to soothe the digestive tract and prevent inflammation within the digestive system. When combined with cows' milk, it can make the milk easier to digest and can be used to help clear coughs. Turmeric can be used in other ways to treat coughs, but combining it with milk works well, as it reduces the milk's tendency to create excess mucus or *kapha*, while the milk softens the excessively drying nature of turmeric. Excessive consumption can be drying and heating, so use with caution.

External use Turmeric can be made into a poultice (see page 96). Note that turmeric has been used to make dyes – it is likely to stain fabrics it comes into contact with and will leave your skin with a yellow hue (this will fade over a short period of time).

A note on water

For the infusions and decoctions in this section, use filtered water if you have it. Otherwise, use regular tap water. Avoid bottled water due to its high carbon footprint.

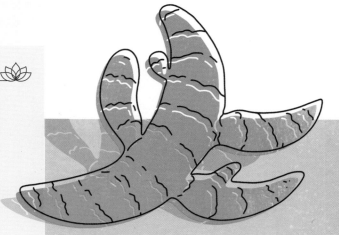

Lemon and Turmeric Pain Poultice

This is a wonderful treatment for arthritic conditions, especially when there is some swelling and pain, particularly around the joints (but not burning heat sensations). It helps to alleviate inflammation, stiffness and pain, and is great for easing pain associated with frozen shoulder and plantar fasciitis. In Ayurveda it is known as *Jambeera pinda sweda*. To apply the poultice, you will need 1 piece of muslin (cheesecloth), 20 × 20cm (8 × 8in), and 1 elastic band, piece of string or strip of fabric. Gently massage the poultice into the troubled area, or hold the poultice against it, for 5–10 minutes or until it feels as though it has penetrated the body. Wash the area with warm water and soap afterwards to remove the turmeric.

Makes 1 application

1 tablespoon coconut oil
1 whole lemon, roughly chopped (including the peel)
1 tablespoon ground unrefined salt
1 tablespoon turmeric

Heat the coconut oil in a frying pan set over a medium heat. Add the chopped lemon and lightly fry for 5–6 minutes, until the skin begins to soften. Mix in the salt and turmeric, cook for another minute, then take the pan off the heat.

Place the mixture into the centre of the muslin square. Gather the edges of the fabric around the poultice to encase it tightly, then secure them with an elastic band or string to enclose the mixture as a compact mass. Allow the mixture to cool enough to handle safely before using.

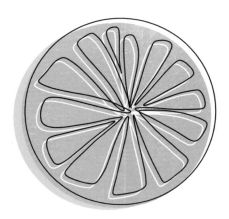

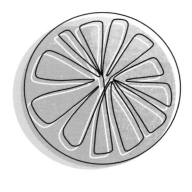

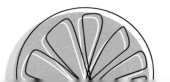

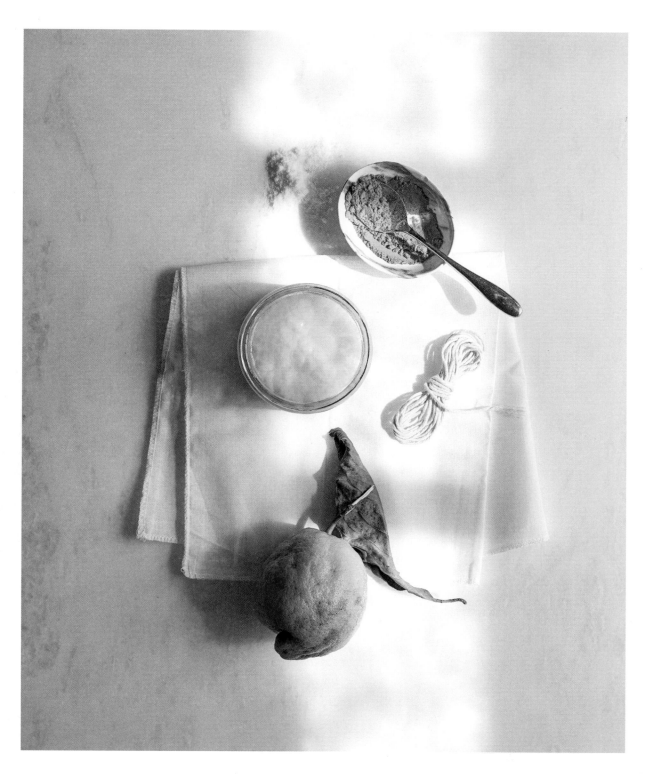

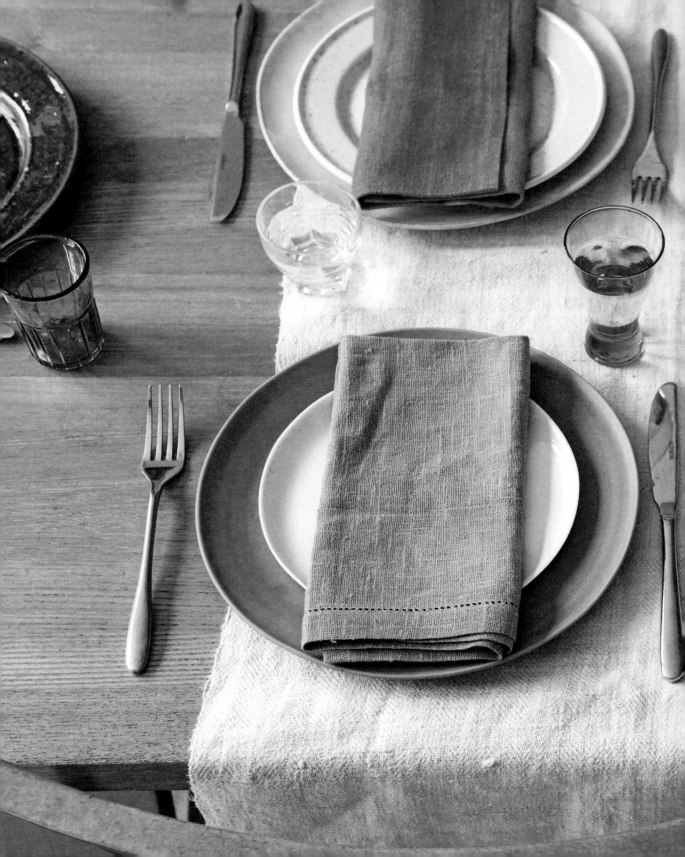

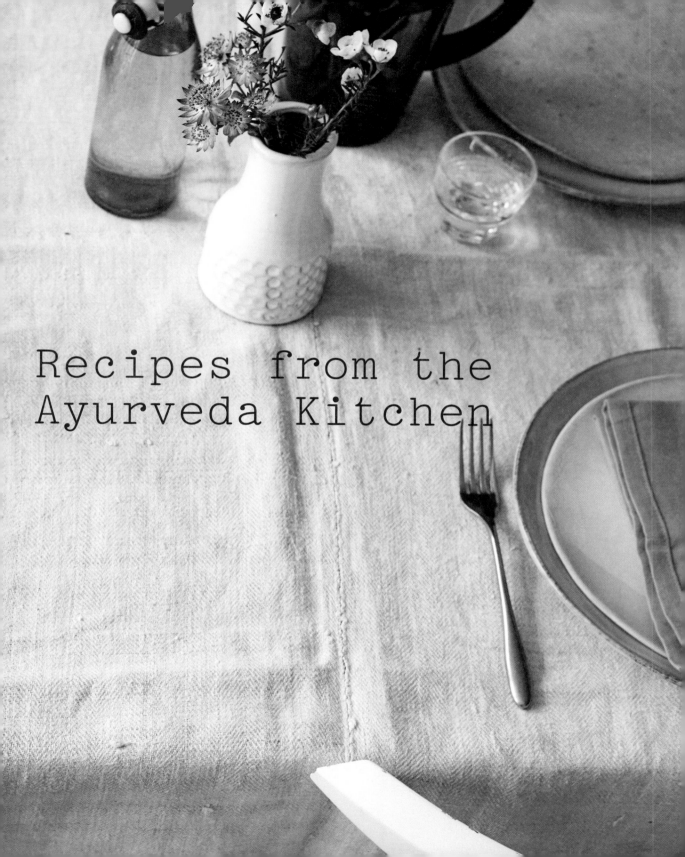

Recipes from the
Ayurveda Kitchen

Breakfast

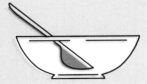

Breakfast is important as it stokes the digestive fire (see page 18) for the rest of the day. When possible, your first meal should be eaten at the same time each day and the quantity should be enough to make you feel full. We are all individual in our body shape and activities so if you find the portion sizes are not right for you, feel free to adjust them.

These Ayurveda-inspired breakfasts will give you energy until lunchtime without the need for a mid-morning snack. This way, when you get to lunch, your body will have secreted the right amount of digestive juices to take care of the meal, leaving no unwanted metabolic waste (see page 20).

I have written many of these recipes with a yield of one portion, as so many of us usually prepare breakfast for one. If you are cooking for family and friends, simply multiply the quantities as necessary.

In some cases, I suggest soaking ingredients such as porridge oats, oat bran, amaranth, nuts and dried fruits overnight in cold water, which removes their drying effects on the body, allowing them instead to have a more harmonizing action. If pre-soaking is too much to contemplate, bear in mind it is better to skip that step and eat the dishes without soaking than to avoid them totally. If you do have the time and inclination, you will be amazed at the difference soaking makes, producing a lighter, fluffier and more wholesome flavour and texture.

There are both savoury and sweet breakfast options included in this section. If the only savoury breakfast you have tried is the traditional Western fry-up, I would urge you to give my alternatives a go and see how you feel after a few days of eating a different kind of savoury breakfast.

If you like to kick-start your day with a caffeinated tea or coffee, Ayurveda is not against this. Everything can be enjoyed in moderation, so have one with your breakfast, but perhaps consider cutting back on additional cups later in the day. Full-fat organic milk helps to balance the drying effect of tannins in black tea and the stimulating effects of coffee. Otherwise, explore the world of herbal teas, or simply drink straight-up hot water, which promotes good digestion and hydrates the body well, especially the colon.

Breathing exercise

This short but effective breathing exercise can be done in your kitchen every morning in order to initiate a healthy breathing pattern, posture and metabolism for the day ahead. You could perhaps practise it while your breakfast is cooking and feel free to incorporate it into your kitchen experience at different times of the day, such as when standing at the kitchen counter after a busy day, before you start to prepare your evening meal. All breathing is done through the nose if possible.

Preparation

Stand with your feet hip-width apart, with a soft bend in the knees. Lift your toes, stretch and spread them out. Now as you return them to the floor, claw at it with the tips of your toes and engage the arches of your feet. Now relax the toes. Feel yourself lifting up through your legs. Lift your chest slightly and drop your shoulders. Take a couple of smooth, long breaths. Place your hands on your ribcage. Take a gentle elongated breath and feel your ribcage moving outward.

Exercise sequence

Observe the path the breath takes. At the end of your next exhalation, engage the pelvic floor muscles, draw the stomach muscles in toward the spine and move the chin subtly backward toward the neck. Hold momentarily and, when the body naturally seeks to inhale, gently release the muscles and let a new breath flow into the body. Repeat this breathing sequence 3–5 times. By the fifth breath you may notice your natural breaths have become longer and your nasal passages are clearer, and that you are feeling a little brighter.

Summertime mineral-boosting yogurt _____

You get lots of minerals in one delicious bowl with this dish. It also promotes good intestinal flora. The warming ginger ensures that the digestive fire (see page 18) is there to take up the minerals. Yogurt is both cooling (from its heavy, moist nature) and heating (from its fermentation process). Have this breakfast during late spring, summer and early autumn, when the weather is warmer and the cooling nature of yogurt is desirable, especially first thing in the morning, when the temperature is naturally colder outside.

Serves 1
Preparation time 5 minutes

4 dried figs
4 dried prunes
handful of raisins
100ml (3½fl oz) water
100ml (3½fl oz) organic full-fat yogurt
tiny pinch of ground ginger

Put the dried fruits into a bowl, cover with the measured water and leave to soak overnight.

In the morning, remove the stones from the prunes, if there are any, then tip the soaking fruits, plus the soaking water, into the jug of a blender. Blend to a liquid consistency, then stir in the yogurt. It really is that easy! If you do not have a blender, mash the softened fruits in a bowl with the back of a fork and slowly add in the yogurt, continuing to mash until the mixture has a homogenous consistency.

Transfer the mixture to a bowl to serve.

Tip
If you are constipated, eating this dish can help to facilitate bowel movements.

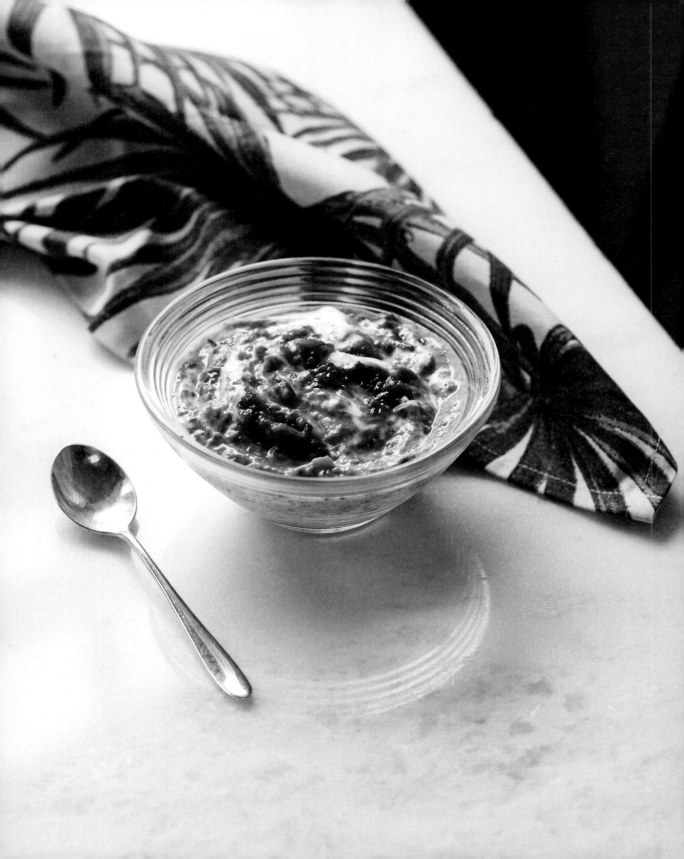

Alchemical oat porridge

As this porridge cooks, the kitchen is filled with its warming, spicy aroma, igniting your taste buds to get you gently salivating first thing in the morning. It is a hearty and warming bowl to start your days with, especially during cooler seasons. I have had countless clients who have started every day with this porridge for years and reaped the benefits. The cinnamon, cardamom and ginger help to warm the body and gently enhance digestive capacity, but they can be omitted if you do not like their flavours. Almonds give good lustre to the skin and are supportive to reproductive tissues.

Serves 1
Preparation time 5 minutes, plus soaking
Cooking time 5 minutes

30g (1oz) porridge oats, soaked overnight
1 tablespoon oat bran, soaked overnight
small handful of raisins, soaked overnight
7 whole almonds, soaked overnight, skins
    removed before using (or use 1 teaspoon
    almond butter)
150ml (¼ pint) boiling water
½ teaspoon ground cinnamon
¼ teaspoon ground cardamom
¼ teaspoon ground ginger

Drain the soaked oats, oat bran, raisins and almonds and put them into a saucepan. Add the measured boiling water, the spices and the almond butter, if using that in place of whole almonds.

Cook the mixture over a medium heat for approximately 5 minutes, stirring occasionally, until cooked. Stir in more boiled water, if you would like the texture of your porridge to be creamier and fluffier, then serve immediately.

Tips

- If you are using unsoaked oats, increase the quantity of water to 200ml (⅓ pint). The cooking time remains roughly the same.

- For those with a sweet tooth, add either a drizzle of maple syrup or ½ teaspoon honey when serving.

- If you find that your bowels can be sluggish, a great way of easing them is to add 1 teaspoon whole linseeds to the cooked porridge as a topping.

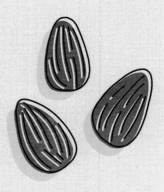

Savoury oat porridge

This savoury porridge is particularly good for keeping your blood sugar balanced from the start of the day. Oats offer slow energy release, allowing you to feel satisfied throughout the morning, and also help to keep bad cholesterol levels down. Try this recipe especially if you tend to feel the cold – sage and thyme are wonderfully warming herbs. Using thyme in cooking during the winter helps to keep the respiratory tract clear. Change the herbs you use in this dish with the seasons for variety of flavour throughout the year.

Serves 1
Preparation time 5 minutes, plus soaking
Cooking time 10 minutes

30g (1oz) porridge oats, soaked overnight
150ml (¼ pint) boiling water
2 thyme sprigs
1 teaspoon olive oil
1 shallot or 3 spring onions, chopped
3 sage leaves
handful of green leaves, such as baby
   spinach, chard and rocket, roughly chopped
unrefined salt and black pepper

To serve
1 teaspoon pumpkin seeds
4 walnut halves

Drain the soaked oats and put them into a saucepan. Add the measured boiling water and 1 of the thyme sprigs and cook over a medium heat, stirring occasionally, for approximately 5 minutes, until cooked.

Meanwhile, heat the oil in a frying pan set over a medium–low heat. Add the shallot or spring onion with the remaining thyme, the sage and the green leaves. Cook gently until the onion is golden – the oats will likely be cooked at this stage as well, but if not, turn off the heat under the onion mixture until the oats are ready.

Once the oats are cooked, check the texture is to your liking – add more water to create a creamy consistency if necessary. With the frying pan off the heat, tip the porridge into the onion and herbs and gently stir to combine. Serve immediately, topped with pumpkin seeds and walnuts.

Tip
If you soak the oats in water overnight, your porridge will be fluffier, tastier and easier to digest. If using unsoaked oats, increase the quantity of water to 200ml (¹/₃ pint). The cooking time remains roughly the same.

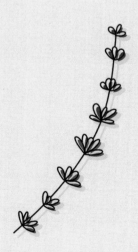

To-go rye and prune breakfast muffins _____

Each mouthful of these wholesome, light, semi-sweet breakfast muffins tastes like a mouthful of goodness. They are packed with fibre, which helps to keep the digestive system healthy. The combination of oats, rye and fruit will sustain you for a long time. Ayurveda considers rye to be astringent and heating, as opposed to the sweet and cooling nature of wheat. Rye contains less gluten than wheat, and lot of soluble fibre, which has positive benefits for the cardiovascular system and the colon, helping to bulk out stools. Helpful gut bacteria love it.

Makes 12–14 muffins
Preparation time 10 minutes
Cooking time 40–45 minutes

few drops of sunflower oil, for greasing
rye flour, for dusting
2 eggs
70ml (2¼fl oz) sunflower oil
175ml (6fl oz) hazelnut milk (see page 190)
2 tablespoons maple syrup
½ teaspoon vanilla paste or seeds from
  ½ vanilla pod
20g (¾oz) sunflower seeds
50g (1¾oz) oats
40g (1½oz) ground hazelnuts
1 dessert apple, peeled, cored and grated
150g (5½oz) pitted prunes, chopped
150g (5½oz) rye flour
1 teaspoon baking powder
¼ teaspoon bicarbonate of soda
70ml (2¼fl oz) water

Preheat the oven to 200°C/180°C fan (400°F), Gas Mark 6. Grease and flour 14 recesses in your muffin tins.

Put the eggs, sunflower oil and hazelnut milk into a bowl and whisk together for a few minutes, until the mixture is frothy. Then, one by one, whisk in the remaining ingredients in the order listed, ensuring each addition is fully incorporated before adding the next.

Spoon a heaped tablespoon of the batter into each recess of the prepared muffin tin. Bake for 40–45 minutes, until cooked through. Leave to cool in the tin for a few minutes, then turn out the muffins onto a wire rack. Serve warm, or leave to cool completely and store in an airtight container for up to 3 days.

Tips
• These muffins are handy when you need to take breakfast with you, and are also great for when you have been working hard physically and need a mid-morning or mid-afternoon energy boost.

• If you are using your own homemade hazelnut milk to make these muffins (see page 190), you can use 40g (1½oz) of the left-over pulp in place of the ground hazelnuts in this recipe.

• Use any type of oats for making these muffins. If you use rolled oats, they will be more prominent after baking. Porridge oats would produce a smoother consistency.

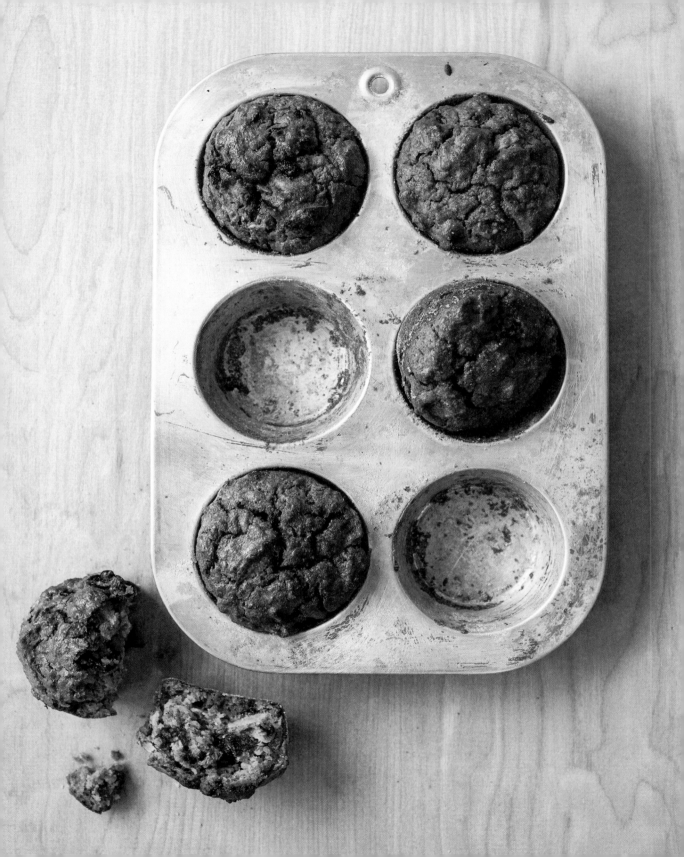

Multi-grain muesli

This muesli contains a range of grains, so is balancing for every constitutional type (see page 15) and promotes good bowel habits. Grains can be challenging for some digestive systems, so adding natural yogurt boosts the intestinal flora and aids the digestion process. Feel free to use whichever grains, seeds and nuts you can get hold of or feel like eating for this recipe. The joy of making your own muesli is that you can include the exact ingredients that you like. So, if you love hazelnuts for example, throw some in.

Makes 8 servings
Preparation time 2 minutes

100g (3½oz) porridge oats
100g (3½oz) barley flakes
100g (3½oz) rice flakes
10g (¼oz) linseeds
10g (¼oz) sunflowers seeds
10g (¼oz) wheatgerm
25g (1oz) flaked almonds
50g (1¾oz) raisins
1 tablespoon ground cinnamon
yogurt or water, to serve

Mix everything together and store in an airtight container for up to six months.

Serving muesli with cold milk poured on top is not the ideal way of eating it, because cold milk cools the digestive system, which can make it harder to digest, potentially leading to excessive gas, bloating or mucus production. What is more, the unsoftened raw grains are considered abrasive to the digestive system. It is preferable, in the warmer months, to soak the muesli overnight in water or yogurt and enjoy it at room temperature in the morning. Alternatively, pour some boiling water over the grains in the morning and allow them to soften for around 5 minutes. The grains will still have a slight bite, but will be much easier to digest. If you want to add some yogurt, do so after the boiling water has worked its magic.

Tip
This muesli can also be cooked into a delicious porridge very easily. Soak 40g (1½oz) of the muesli in water overnight and follow the Alchemical Oat Porridge recipe on page 104.

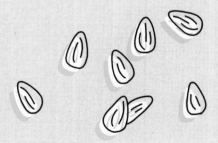

Fruit compote

For those with a lighter morning appetite, this is the ideal breakfast. Fruit compotes provide a fresh-tasting meal. They can be made the night before and reheated in the morning if you are short of time. Either of the suggested fruits tastes lovely. Pears are sweet and grounding. Apples are also sweet, but sour and astringent as well, therefore promoting a lighter quality than pears. Other seasonal fruits can be added or substituted, depending on the fruit – I like rhubarb (add a little coconut sugar or maple syrup), blackberries and raspberries.

Serves 1
Preparation time 3 minutes
Cooking time 7 minutes

2 dessert apples or pears, cored and
   roughly chopped
50ml (2fl oz) water
3 cloves
½ teaspoon ground ginger
½ teaspoon ground cinnamon
½ teaspoon ghee (see page 196; optional)

Put the pieces of fruit into a saucepan with the measured water, spices and ghee, if using. Simmer gently over a medium–low heat until the fruit breaks down to a mushy consistency. This will take approximately 7 minutes, depending on the ripeness of the fruit – soft pear cooks far more quickly than apple.

Transfer the compote to a bowl, discard the cloves and serve immediately, or leave to cool, then store in an airtight container in the refrigerator for 2–3 days. To reheat, place the compote in a saucepan and bring to simmering point, then heat gently over a low heat for 2 minutes, stirring occasionally, until heated through – stir in a splash of water if it looks too thick.

Tips

- If you find that your skin is particularly dry, I would advise you add the optional ghee when making this dish.

- If, after eating this for breakfast, you find that you are ravenous mid-morning, this suggests that fruits alone are not enough to sustain you until lunchtime. Consider topping the compote with some nuts and seeds – try walnuts, almonds, sunflower seeds and pumpkin seeds. If you are still hungry by mid-morning, I suggest switching to a grain-based breakfast.

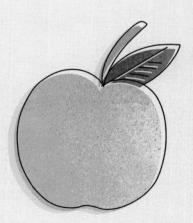

Soda bread

This soda bread is ideal for sharing. According to Ayurveda, rye flour is good for those who are a little heavier, while wheat flour is appropriate for those who are lighter. Combining the two flours in this bread makes it suitable for most people, especially since yeast, which can cause digestive disturbances in some people, is omitted. Soda bread is denser than leavened bread, a tasty loaf in its own way. The combination of rye and wholemeal flours produces a wholesome taste, and the close grain has a nice texture.

Serves 4–6
Preparation time 2 minutes
Cooking time 30–35 minutes

125g (4½oz) wholemeal flour
125g (4½oz) rye flour
2 teaspoons cream of tartar
1 teaspoon bicarbonate of soda
pinch of unrefined salt
200ml (⅓ pint) water
1 teaspoon olive oil
nut butters, honey, olive oil or pesto, to serve

Preheat the oven to 200°C/180°C fan (400°F), Gas Mark 6. Line a baking sheet with baking paper.

Combine the dry ingredients in a bowl, then stir in the measured water using a fork (try to be as light-handed as possible, to keep as much air in the mixture in order to produce a lighter loaf), until the mixture forms a soft dough. Add the olive oil and lightly fold it in.

Plop the sloppy dough onto the centre of the prepared baking sheet. Trying to retain some height in the dough ball, gently smooth out the top with the back of a knife, then use the knife to score a criss-cross pattern onto the top of the loaf to mark out 6 servings. Transfer immediately to the oven and bake for 30–35 minutes, until the bread sounds hollow when knocked on its base.

Serve warm with nut butters, honey, olive oil or pesto, or transfer to a wire rack and leave to cool. Soda bread does not stay fresh for long and should be enjoyed on the day of baking.

Tip
Many people have a psychological block when it comes to preparing a cooked breakfast, believing it will be too time-consuming. The blessing with this recipe is that it is so quick and easy to prepare, there is virtually no excuse not to make it. You can quickly put it together and get it in the oven to cook while you are preparing for the day ahead, then start your day with a warming, nourishing breakfast.

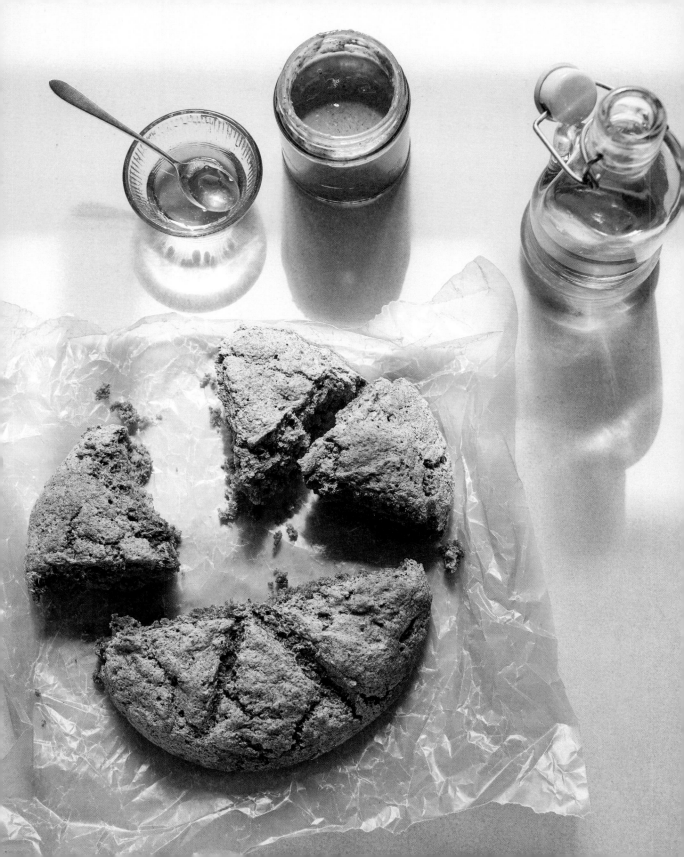

Buckwheat pancakes

For those who find wheat difficult to digest, buckwheat flour offers a great alternative – buckwheat is a member of the rhubarb family, which means it is gluten-free. It has a more complex taste than wheat. Buckwheat is astringent, sweet and heating, and helps to prevent mucus build up, so these pancakes are ideal for days when the weather is extremely damp and cold. They provide a real breakfast treat, especially when made with maple syrup.

Serves 2 (makes 4 pancakes)
Preparation time 2 minutes
Cooking time 15–20 minutes

50g (1¾oz) buckwheat flour
100ml (3½fl oz) almond milk (see page 190)
1 egg
2–4 teaspoons ghee (see page 196) or
  sunflower oil

Sweet option
2 tablespoons maple syrup
½ teaspoon ground cinnamon
fresh berries, fruit compote or honey, to serve

Savoury option
tiny pinch of turmeric (or use a 1cm/½in
  piece of fresh turmeric, peeled and grated)
nut butter or fresh herbs with a little grated
  cheese, to serve

Put the flour, milk and egg into a large bowl. If making the sweet option, add the maple syrup and cinnamon. If making the savoury option, add the turmeric. Whisk to form a smooth batter.

Heat a frying pan for 1–2 minutes over a medium–high heat, until it is hot enough for cooking the pancakes. To test if the pan is ready, splash a few droplets of water onto it – if they jump and fizz, the pan is ready.

Heat ½ teaspoon ghee or sunflower oil in a frying pan over a high heat for a few seconds, then lower the heat to medium and pour in a quarter of the batter. Tilt the pan from side to side to encourage the batter to spread and thinly cover the base of the pan. Cook for 1–2 minutes, until bubbles form on the surface and the edges lift up slightly from the base of the pan. At this point, turn the pancake over and cook for 1–2 minutes more, until it is golden on both sides. If your pancakes begin to stick you may need to add ½ teaspoon more oil to the pan. Transfer to a warmed plate and keep warm while you cook the remaining pancakes. Serve immediately, with sweet or savoury toppings, as desired.

Tips
• When the weather is dry or you feel like a treat, add the sweet additions to the batter for a delicious treat. When the weather is inclement, turmeric is the more suitable option.

• These pancakes can be prone to sticking to the pan. Ensure your pan is well seasoned and heated to a high temperature before adding the oil. I would only ever recommend using a nonstick pan when cooking pancakes, but a well-seasoned regular pan should work fine and is preferable from a health perspective.

Breakfast protein pot

This breakfast dish is brimming with goodness and is particularly useful to vegetarians and vegans due to its high protein content. Amaranth is a lesser-known grain that is packed with protein, and wheatgerm promotes good brain functioning. The almond adds extra protein and the cinnamon helps to metabolize it all. All together it has a nice nutty bite.

Serves 1
Preparation time 1 minute, plus soaking
Cooking time 20–30 minutes

40g (1½oz) amaranth, soaked overnight
1 tablespoon wheatgerm
pinch of ground cinnamon
250ml (9fl oz) boiling water
1 teaspoon almond butter
1 teaspoon raisins
1 teaspoon sunflower seeds

Drain the soaked amaranth and put it into a saucepan with the wheatgerm, cinnamon and measured boiling water. Bring to the boil, then simmer the amaranth over a medium heat for 20–30 minutes, until light and fluffy. Stir in the almond butter at the end of cooking.

Transfer the spiced amaranth to a bowl, top with the raisins and sunflower seeds and serve immediately.

Tip
Getting the consistency of this porridge right can be tricky to begin with, but it is worth persevering, as this dish is so nutritious. Just keep tasting and stirring. After about 20 minutes, the mixture will suddenly come together into a porridge consistency, and the tiny grains will taste a little nutty on the outside and be soft in the middle. Add more water if it looks as though the mixture is drying out.

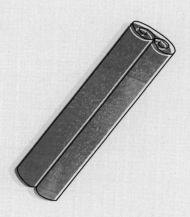

Sustaining savoury rice bowl ————————————

Like oat porridge, this rice dish is very sustaining throughout the morning. Garlic is great for cardiovascular health, especially when consumed first thing in the morning, as is ginger, for digestive health. Seaweed is very high in iodine, promoting good thyroid functioning; eaten first thing in the morning, it can stoke the metabolic fire for the rest of the day. Make the dish with quinoa if you fancy some variety.

Serves 1
Preparation time 5 minutes
Cooking time 10 minutes

½ teaspoon olive oil or ghee (see page 196)
1 garlic clove, chopped
pinch of turmeric
1cm (½in) piece of fresh root ginger,
    chopped
handful of green leaves, such as spinach,
    rocket and watercress
125g (4½oz) cooked rice (or use cooked
    quinoa instead)
tamari soy sauce
sprinkle of seaweed flakes
1 teaspoon sesame seeds

Heat the oil or ghee gently in a saucepan, then add the garlic, turmeric and ginger and fry over a low heat for 4–5 minutes, until the garlic and ginger are soft.

Toss in the green leaves, followed by the rice. Mix in some tamari to taste, then stir in the seaweed and sesame seeds. Cook for 2–3 minutes, until the rice or quinoa is heated through, then serve immediately.

Tip
This dish makes a good lunch too, so double the quantities and prepare an extra batch. Put that, hot from the pan, straight into a flask for lunch, adding extra vegetables if desired.

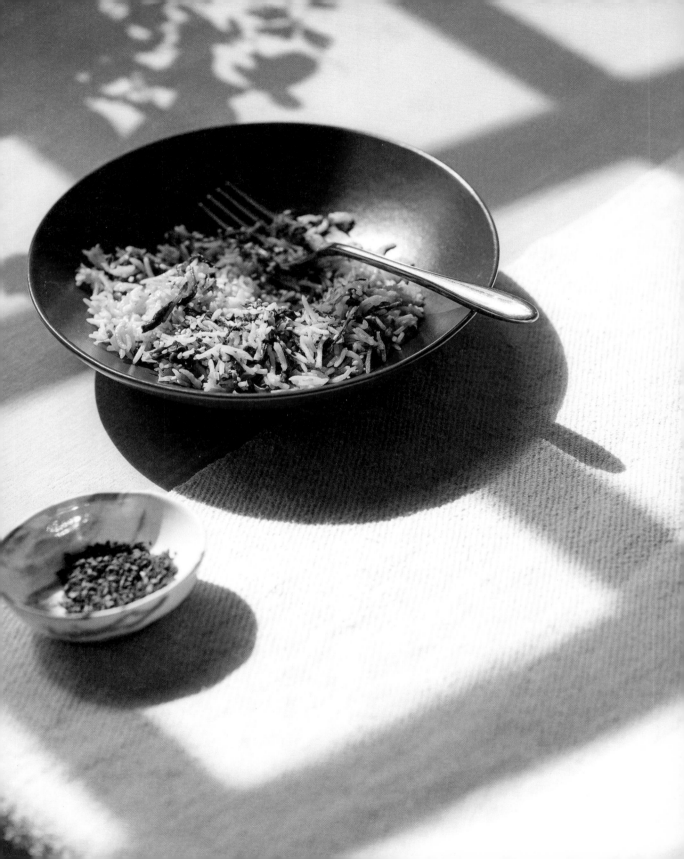

Morning kitchen energy

Understanding our natural biorhythms helps to guide us in
how to operate in our kitchens in the morning. Some of us
naturally feel chirpier in the morning than others, but on
the whole, our circadian rhythms are the same and are closely
linked to sunlight.

With the sun's rays streaming into our kitchens from the
sky at a low angle, the light and feeling within our kitchens
is different to that of other times of day. The soundscape
differs too: the sounds the weather causes; the dawn chorus;
the background sounds of heating pipes; showers running in
the distance. This morning atmosphere of the kitchen mirrors
our internal waking up. The climatic conditions of the day
will always influence, to a degree, how we move around our
kitchens and what we choose to prepare for breakfast. Just as
you would plan to wear a jumper if it is looking cold outside,
so you may decide to cook something warmer. So, when you wake
up, have a good look outside, connect with what nature is
offering up for the day and plan your meals accordingly.

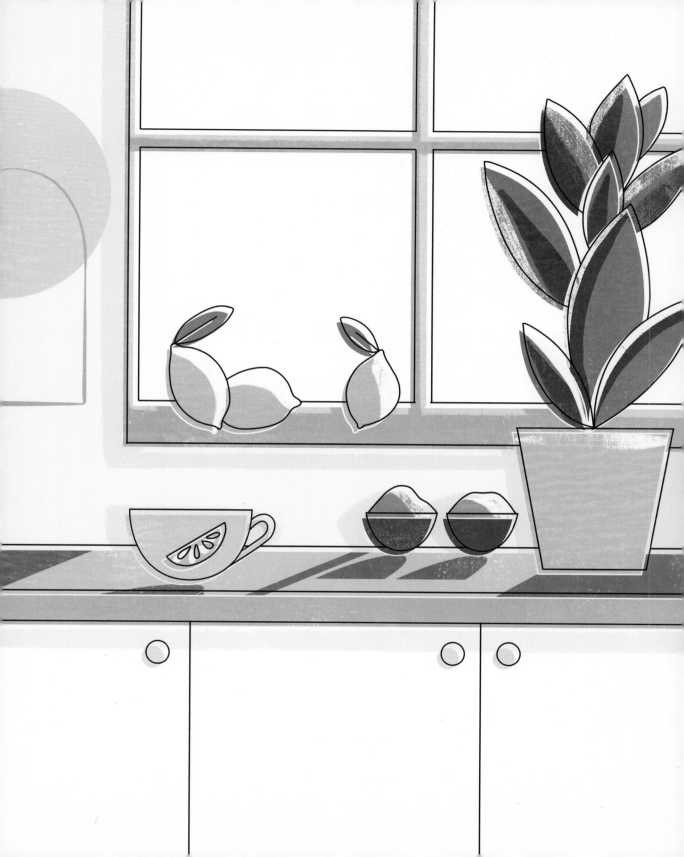

Lunch

From an Ayurvedic perspective, lunch should be the biggest meal of the day. This is because our bodies have a higher digestive capacity at lunchtime, which means the meal is digested most easily and the optimum nutritive properties of the food are absorbed. Eating a large meal late at night, when the body's natural digestive capacity is lower, can lead to sluggishness and lethargy the next day. However, this pattern of eating can be difficult to achieve in the modern world, owing to cultural norms and working patterns.

The recipes that many people would normally have in the evening have instead been placed within the lunch section of this book to emphasize the significance of lunch as the main meal of the day. If you are at home at lunchtime, this may be achievable. Certainly, if you work from home, it will be easier as, with many of the recipes, if you can factor in the preparation time, you can then leave the dish to cook and slowly continue with your work.

However, if you are unable to be at home for lunch, taking a larger pre-cooked meal with you to work may be a good option – in which case, the dedicated Packed Lunch section (see pages 134–47) will offer you guidance. Otherwise, if you decide to use any of the lunch recipes in the evening, enjoy slightly smaller portions and try not to eat too close to bedtime.

Post-lunch exercise

The very best exercise after lunch has to be a brisk walk.
This is by far the most beneficial thing you can do for your
digestive system, your mental fitness and overall wellbeing.
It will help you to prevent a mid-afternoon slump from
the digestive system being sluggish, and you should feel
revitalized ahead of the afternoon's activities. A ten-minute
brisk walk is ideal, but even five minutes will suffice if
that is all the time you have. While you are walking, bear
in mind the following points:

- engage your arms, moving them backward and forward as
  you walk

- consciously drop your shoulders and relax your neck muscles
  if you have excessively stiffened them

- practise diaphragmatic breathing (see page 44) and allow
  your breath to become more expansive

- do not stare at the ground in front of you as you walk or
  become so engrossed in your thoughts you fail to see the
  world around you. Instead, connect with nature and the
  environment you are walking through

- keep any mobile phones or other devices firmly in your
  pocket and avoid the temptation to be busy with other
  things at this time

- engage your senses as you walk, becoming aware of the
  sounds, smells and sights you encounter. You may find
  something inspiring and uplifting to carry into the
  afternoon with you.

Light and simple pak choi and noodle stir-fry _____

The components of the Chinese five-spice blend act as both appetizers and digestants, meaning they help at all stages of digestion. This dish is ideal for when you are feeling sluggish and need to cleanse the body of lingering waste matter, or when the weather is damp and cold.

Serves 2
Preparation time 10 minutes
Cooking time 10 minutes

1 teaspoon sunflower oil
1 teaspoon Chinese five-spice
1cm (½in) piece of fresh root ginger, peeled and roughly chopped
1 garlic clove, diced
1 green pepper, cored, deseeded and sliced into strips
10cm (4in) piece of cucumber, cut into strips
1 celery stick, cut into strips
2 heads of pak choi or spring greens, roughly chopped
1 teaspoon tamari soy sauce
200g (7oz) rice or soba noodles
1 tablespoon chopped seaweed salad
1 tablespoon sesame seeds
handful of cashew nuts

Heat the sunflower oil in a wok over a low heat, then add the five-spice, followed by the ginger, garlic and green pepper, and cook for 2–3 minutes, until the spice aromas are released. Then add the cucumber, celery, pak choi and tamari. Fry gently for 3–4 minutes, until slightly soft. If the vegetables become too dry, add a little splash of water.

Meanwhile, cook the noodles according to the packet instructions.

Add the cooked noodles, seaweed salad, sesame seeds and cashew nuts to the wok and toss together to serve.

Tip
This dish is delicious eaten hot or cold. Transfer the freshly cooked stir-fry directly to a food flask in the winter, or allow to cool before you put it in a plastic storage container in the summer, for a tasty packed lunch.

120

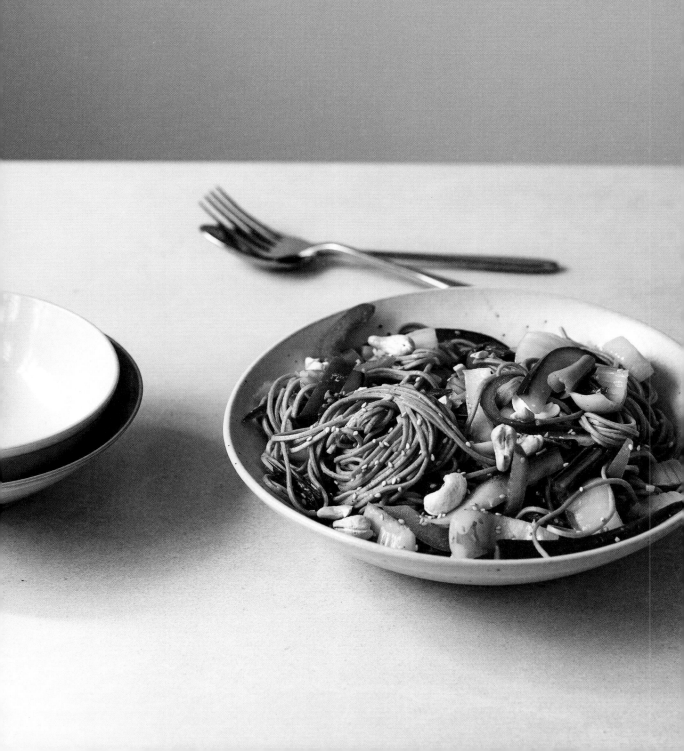

Vegetarian paella _____

Saffron is balancing for all constitutional types (see page 15) and also very rejuvenating. This wonderful spice is cooling, while sweet paprika is gently heating, so the two counterbalance each other and enhance the flavour of the rice.

Serves 4–5
Preparation time 7 minutes
Cooking time 55–60 minutes

1 tablespoon olive oil
2 sweet pointed or red peppers, cored, deseeded and sliced lengthways
1 onion, finely diced
2 garlic cloves, finely diced
1 litre (1¾ pints) vegetable stock
pinch of saffron threads
1 fennel bulb, thinly sliced horizontally
splash of sherry or white wine
2 teaspoons sweet paprika
1 tablespoon chopped seaweed salad
350g (12oz) paella rice
3 handfuls of fresh broad beans or peas (or use frozen)
unrefined salt and black pepper

To garnish
handful of flat leaf parsley, chopped
1 lemon, cut into wedges

Heat the oil in a paella pan or very large frying pan over a medium–low heat. Add the pepper and cook for 3–4 minutes, until it begins to soften and colour, then stir in the onion and garlic and cook gently for 5 minutes or so, until the onion is translucent.

Meanwhile, bring the vegetable stock to a boil in a saucepan over a high heat, then reduce the heat to low to simmer the stock. Stir the saffron strands into the hot stock so they begin to release their flavour into it, turn off the heat and leave the saffron to infuse the stock.

When the garlic and onion in the paella pan are soft, stir in the fennel and cook for a further 3 minutes, until the fennel begins to soften. Stir in a splash of sherry or white wine and cook for 2 minutes or so to allow most of it to evaporate. Then mix in the sweet paprika and seaweed salad, and season with salt and pepper. Add the rice and combine it thoroughly with the other ingredients, then spread it out evenly across the base of the pan. Finally, pour over the hot saffron stock.

Leave to cook over a medium heat for 40 minutes or so, until all the stock is absorbed and the rice is cooked. After the first few minutes of cooking, gently move some of the rice around in the pan to ensure it is evenly distributed. After this, check the pan regularly and add up to 50ml (2fl oz) water at a time if the mixture starts to become dry. Approximately 7 minutes before the end of the cooking time, add the broad beans or peas, pushing them into the rice so they cook through.

Serve the paella sprinkled with chopped parsley, with lemon wedges alongside.

Tip
Seaweed salad combines a variety of finely chopped seaweeds. If you are unable to source any, use finely chopped sheet nori or simply omit the seaweed.

Puy lentil and nut roast

Lentils are astringent and heating, while oats are sweet and cooling, so they balance each other perfectly in this dish. Walnuts are full of manganese, which is essential for healthy bones. In Ayurveda, walnuts are considered to be a tonic for the nervous system. This dish is delicious served with some steamed seasonal vegetables and gravy.

Serves 2–3
Preparation time 5 minutes, plus soaking
Cooking time 20–30 minutes

125g (4½oz) dried Puy lentils, soaked for at least 4 hours, cooked according to the packet instructions (reserve 4 tablespoons cooking water for mashing)
60g (2¼oz) porridge oats
2 tablespoons olive oil
½ teaspoon garlic salt
½ teaspoon sweet paprika
pinch of black pepper
3 teaspoons freshly chopped sage and lemon balm, or dried mixed herbs
60g (2¼oz) walnuts, roughly chopped
2 tablespoons grated hard cheese (optional)

Preheat the oven to 200°C/180°C fan (400°F), Gas Mark 6. Line a 450g (1lb) loaf tin with baking paper.

Put the cooked lentils into a large bowl with the reserved cooking water and mash them. Add the remaining ingredients, except the cheese, and stir together.

Spoon the mixture into the prepared loaf tin, sprinkle over the grated cheese, if desired, then bake for 20–30 minutes, until firm and slightly browned. Leave to cool in the tin for 5 minutes.

Tip out the lentil and nut roast carefully onto a chopping board, then cut it into slices and serve immediately.

Tips
- Any leftover nut roast can be saved for the next day. To reheat, put 1 teaspoon olive oil or ½ teaspoon ghee into a small frying pan, add the nut roast to the pan and fry gently, stirring it around to heat it through.

- If you like the taste of horseradish, it works very well alongside this nut roast.

- Brown or green lentils can be substituted for Puy lentils in this dish. If you wish to use canned lentils, use a 400g (14oz) can, drain and wash the lentils, and use regular water for mashing.

- If using grated hard cheese, switching the type you use each time you make this dish is a great way of keeping things varied. Different cheeses produce such wonderfully different results. For this dish, I might use Manchego one day and a local goats' cheese another time. Use your own preferences as a guide.

Restorative mung bean hotpot

Mung beans are one of the few beans that are easy to digest and are suitable for all constitutional types (see page 15). They do not need to be soaked prior to cooking but, in this dish, I feel it enhances the flavour. Thyme and bay are both gently heating herbs and support the respiratory system. If you want to serve something alongside, try it with some steamed green vegetables.

Serves 2
Preparation time 10 minutes, plus soaking
Cooking time 1½ hours

½ teaspoon ghee (see page 196), plus extra
  for drizzling
2 carrots, peeled and roughly chopped
1 onion, roughly chopped
2 celery sticks, roughly chopped
few dashes of tamari soy sauce
1 tablespoon spelt flour (or use any flour of
  your choice)
100g (3½oz) mung beans, soaked overnight
5 thyme sprigs
2 bay leaves
600ml (20fl oz) hot vegetable stock
2 large potatoes, sliced into rounds
unrefined salt and black pepper

Preheat the oven to 200°C/180°C fan (400°F),
Gas Mark 6.

Heat the ghee in a medium casserole over
a medium–low heat, then stir in the carrot,
onion and celery and fry gently for 5 minutes,
until softened and slightly browned.

Mix in a few dashes of tamari soy sauce, cook
for a further minute or so, then add the flour
and mix well. Now stir in the soaked mung
beans, thyme sprigs and bay leaves and
grind in some black pepper. Add the hot
vegetable stock to the pan, then arrange
the sliced potatoes neatly and gently on top.
Drizzle a little ghee over the potatoes and
season with salt and pepper. Cover the
casserole with a lid, transfer to the oven and
bake for 30 minutes.

Remove the casserole from the oven to check
the mixture is not drying out, and add a dash
of water if necessary. Return the casserole to
the oven and bake for a further 30 minutes.

Remove the lid from the casserole and bake for
a further 15–20 minutes to brown the potato.
Serve immediately.

Tips
- Cooked mung beans or lentils can be
  substituted for minced meat in any recipe.
  Reduce the cooking time, as they will not
  require cooking.

- When soaking the mung beans for this
  dish, soak some extra, so you can sprout
  them over the course of the next few days
  (see pages 68–9).

Goats' cheese, green beans and beetroot couscous _____

Goats' cheese is sour and heating in nature, and has mild potential to increase mucus in the body. In this dish, the pungency of fresh parsley helps to prevent mucus formation. Goats' cheese contains less calcium than cows' cheese, but it is easier to digest. Goats' milk is astringent, sweet and cold, whereas cow's milk is just sweet and cold.

Serves 1
Preparation time 10 minutes
Cooking time 35 minutes

1 large beetroot, peeled and cut into
   small dice
1 teaspoon ghee (see page 196)
1 leek, chopped
handful of green beans
30g (1oz) goats' cheese
small handful of fresh flat-leaf parsley,
   roughly chopped

For the couscous
75g (2¾oz) wheat or barley couscous
100ml (3½fl oz) boiling water
1 tablespoon olive oil
2 tablespoons lemon juice
unrefined salt and black pepper

Boil the beetroot for approximately 30 minutes, until soft.

Gently heat the ghee in a saucepan set over a medium–low heat. Add the leek, green beans, cooked beetroot and a splash of water, cover with a lid and cook gently for around 5 minutes, until the leek is cooked and the green beans are tender.

While the vegetables are cooking, put the couscous into a small bowl, pour over the boiling water, then cover with a side plate to trap the steam. Leave to stand for 5 minutes to allow the grain to absorb all the water, then remove the plate and use a fork to fluff up the couscous. Taste the couscous to see if it is fully cooked – if not, add a little more water, replace the plate and leave for a little longer. Once you are satisfied it is cooked, drizzle over the olive oil and lemon juice, season with salt and pepper, and mix well.

Once the vegetables are cooked, crumble the goats' cheese over them and allow it to melt slightly, then sprinkles with the parsley.

Serve the couscous warm, topped with the cooked vegetables.

Tips
• This dish is suited to summer and early autumn, when beans and beetroot are in season. It is like a warm salad – perfectly suited to the climate at this time of year.

• The beetroot can be cooked in advance. Leave it to cool, then store it in the fridge until you are ready to prepare the dish.

Satisfying black-eyed bean burgers _____

These burgers are great for vegetarians, as the combination of quinoa and black-eyed beans provides a complementary plant protein, to maximize your protein uptake. Beans contain a lot of soluble and insoluble fibre. Both are essential for a healthy gut. Insoluble fibre in particular feeds certain gut bacteria, leading to a good digestive fire. Meat eaters will love these burgers too – they offer a hugely satisfying meal. Serve the burgers with this herby quinoa, some steamed seasonal vegetables, such as corn on the cob as summer slides into autumn, or purple sprouting broccoli during spring, and a dollop of Ginger, Red Cabbage and Beetroot Sauerkraut (see page 194).

Serves 2
Preparation time 10 minutes, plus soaking
Cooking time 1 hour

100g (3½oz) black-eyed beans, soaked
   overnight (or use 400g/14oz canned
   black-eyed beans)
1½ teaspoons ghee (see page 196) or
   sunflower oil
pinch of cumin seeds, lightly crushed
1 onion, finely diced
1 small garlic clove, finely diced
handful of spinach, roughly chopped
1 tablespoon wholemeal flour

For the quinoa
60g (2¼oz) quinoa, soaked overnight
1 teaspoon olive oil
1 teaspoon lemon juice
1 teaspoon chopped seasonal herbs,
   such as mint, oregano or parsley
unrefined salt and black pepper

Cook the soaked black-eyed beans according to the packet instructions (this takes approximately 45 minutes) until they are soft. Then drain and set aside.

While the beans are cooking, heat ½ teaspoon of the ghee in a frying pan over a medium–low heat, then add the crushed cumin seeds and fry gently for a few moments to release their aroma. Stir in the onion and cook for 5 minutes or so, until softened. Add the garlic and spinach and sauté for a further 2 minutes, until the spinach has wilted.

Take the frying pan off the heat and stir in the cooked beans (or drained and rinsed canned beans). Set the mixture aside until it has cooled a little.

Meanwhile, cook the quinoa according to the packet instructions. It is ready when the little 'tails' uncurl and the grains are soft but still retain some bite.

While the quinoa is cooking, shape and fry the burgers. Once the bean mixture is cool enough to handle, mash it slightly (leave some texture in the mixture), adding 1–2 tablespoons water to help it bind, if necessary. Sprinkle the flour onto a plate. Using wet hands, shape half the bean mixture into a patty. Gently toss the patty in the flour, then set to one side and use the remaining bean mixture to form a second patty in the same way.

Heat the remaining ghee or sunflower oil in a clean frying pan over a medium heat, add the patties and lightly fry for 3–4 minutes on each side, until golden brown.

Drain the cooked quinoa if there is any remaining liquid, then return it to the pan with the olive oil and lemon juice. Season with salt and pepper, add the chopped herbs and mix together well. Serve the burgers and quinoa immediately.

Tips

- It is worth making extra bean burgers and quinoa and keeping them in the refrigerator for lunch the next day. In the warmer months, you can put them in a food container in the morning along with some fresh leaves, such as rocket, to eat at room temperature at lunchtime. In the winter, reheat the burgers in the morning and put them into a food flask to eat warm for lunch. To reheat, add ¼ teaspoon ghee to a large heated frying pan, then reduce the heat to medium–low and add the burgers and quinoa, moving them around the pan so they do not stick, until they are warmed through.

- These burgers can be served with other grains, such as couscous or bulgur wheat – the combination of pulse and grain will still provide a complementary protein.

- In Ayurveda, you are advised to avoid canned products owing to their more acid nature. However, if you are time-short and use them sparingly, they provide a useful alternative to dried pulses.

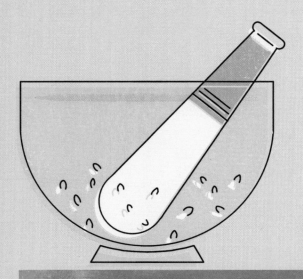

Refreshing edamame beans with roasted butternut squash and red cabbage coleslaw _____

The zingy citrus and crispy crunch of the beans and coleslaw give this meal a refreshing taste. There are no grains served with it, and the edamame beans are well balanced, with ginger and lime counterbalancing any *vata*-inducing qualities of the beans, so it is light on the digestive system. This gives your body the best chance to assimilate all the wonderful nutrients from the edamame beans, in particular the protein. They contain all 9 essential amino acids, making them a high-quality protein source. The bitter, astringent taste of red cabbage comes from anthocyanin compounds, which have high antioxidant activity and help destroy free radicals. These are more bioavailable when cabbage is consumed raw.

Serves 2
Preparation time 20 minutes
Cooking time 35 minutes

For the butternut squash
½ medium-sized butternut squash, peeled and cut into small cubes
½ teaspoon olive oil
unrefined salt and black pepper
small handful of pea shoots, to garnish

For the edamame beans
160g (5¾oz) shelled frozen edamame (soya) beans
½ teaspoon olive oil
¼ teaspoon tamari soy sauce
¼ teaspoon lime juice
1cm (½in) piece of fresh ginger, finely grated
¼ teaspoon finely grated unwaxed lime peel

For the coleslaw
¼ large red cabbage, shredded
1 small fennel bulb, finely sliced
1 small courgette, grated
1 tablespoon olive oil
1 tablespoon lemon juice
2 tablespoons walnut pieces
1 tablespoon pumpkin seeds
unrefined salt and black pepper

Preheat the oven to 200°C/180°C fan (400°F), Gas Mark 6.

Place the butternut squash cubes on a baking tray and drizzle with olive oil and a tablespoon of water. Season with salt and pepper and mix together, then place in the oven to cook for 30 minutes or until the butternut squash cubes begin to brown and caramelize around the edges but remain soft inside. At this point remove them from the oven and allow to cool.

While the squash is cooling, place the edamame beans in a steamer pan and steam for 2 minutes. Remove from the heat, place in a bowl and combine with the other ingredients. In a separate bowl combine the coleslaw ingredients and mix well. Scatter the pea shoots over the butternut squash and serve with the beans and coleslaw.

Tip
Pea shoots are so quick and easy to grow on a windowsill. Simply soak some growing peas in water overnight, then the next day push the peas gently into a pot of compost, water regularly and watch them sprout in 10–18 days. Pea shoots are bursting with *prana* and can be eaten raw.

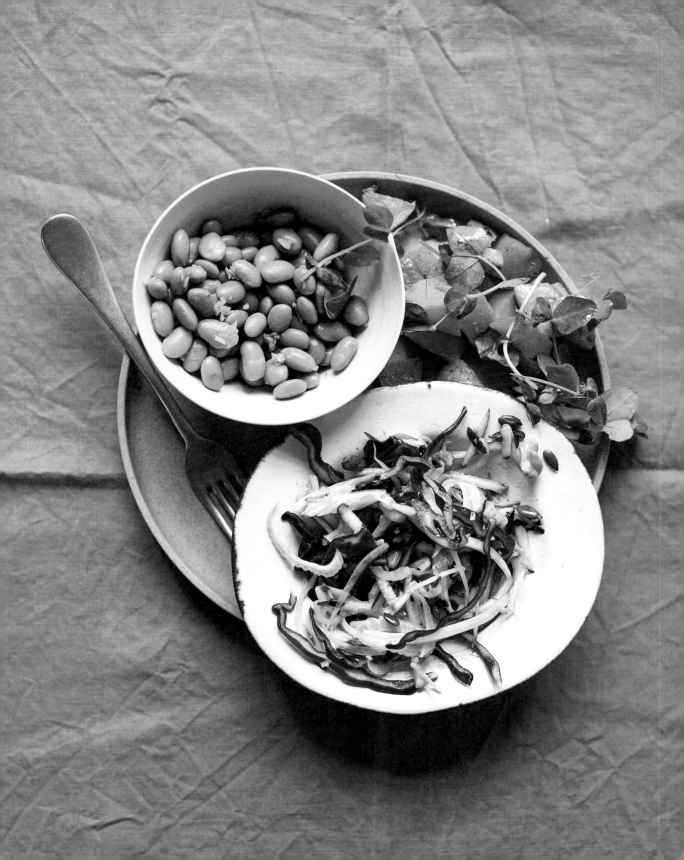

Warming kidney beans with giant couscous _____

Kidney beans are packed with folate, making them an important food for reproduction, blood cell production and cellular health. Soaking overnight helps to unlock the folate. Both the asafoetida and cumin help to minimize the gas-producing potential of the beans. Like most beans, kidney beans are astringent in nature. Serving them with a wheat-based carbohydrate such as giant couscous allows the sweet grain to pacify their astringency. It also helps to create a complementary plant protein combination. The Mexican-style spice mix is gently warming and especially comforting on a cool autumnal day. It goes well with the red cabbage coleslaw on page 128 or some steamed seasonal green vegetables.

Serves 2
Preparation time 10 minutes, plus soaking
Cooking time 1½ hours

For the kidney beans
1 teaspoon olive oil
2 sweet pointed peppers, cored, deseeded
    and thinly sliced lengthways
1 onion, thinly sliced lengthways
1 leek, chopped
3 garlic cloves, quartered
1 teaspoon garlic powder
1 teaspoon sweet paprika
1 teaspoon ground cumin
pinch of asafoetida
1 teaspoon dried oregano
pinch of unrefined rock salt
pinch of black pepper
150g (5½oz) dried kidney beans,
    soaked overnight
1 litre (1¾ pints) water

For the couscous
100g (3½oz) giant couscous
200ml (⅓ pint) water
olive oil, for drizzling
½ lemon
1 tablespoon roughly chopped fresh coriander
1 tablespoon pumpkin seeds
unrefined salt and black pepper

Put all the ingredients for the kidney beans, except the kidney beans and water, into a casserole over a low heat and fry gently for 5 minutes, until the onions start to become translucent. Now stir in the kidney beans and measured water, place the lid on the casserole and simmer over a medium–high heat for 1½ hours, until the kidney beans are tender.

Approximately 20 minutes before the cooking time for the beans has elapsed, place the couscous in a saucepan with the measured water. Bring to a boil, then reduce the heat to medium–low and simmer for 15 minutes, until the couscous is soft. Drain any excess water from the pan, then drizzle with olive oil, squeeze the lemon over and mix in the chopped coriander, pumpkin seeds and some salt and pepper. Serve the kidney beans and couscous immediately.

Tip
If using canned kidney beans, use a 400g (14oz) can. Rinse and drain the beans before use, and reduce the cooking water to 150ml (¼ pint) and cook for only 10 minutes.

Five-spice tofu with rhubarb cabbage _____

Tofu, made from soya beans, has grown in popularity outside of its native China and there are many great products available. Soya beans offer a complete protein with all the essential amino acids that are found in meat and are a good source of iron. Combining tofu with sesame seeds gives it an added calcium kick. It is astringent and sweet, which is balanced out by the warming spices and salty tamari, as well as the sourness of the rhubarb or pomegranate.

Serves 2
Preparation time 15 minutes, plus marinating
Cooking time 10 minutes

For the tofu

200g (7oz) firm tofu, cut into 2cm (¾in) dice
1 tablespoon tamari soy sauce
1 tablespoon sesame seeds
½ teaspoon ghee (see page 196) or olive oil
chives, roughly chopped, to garnish

For the spice mix

2 cloves
½ teaspoon ground cinnamon
1 star anise
½ teaspoon fennel seeds
½ teaspoon black pepper

For the rhubarb cabbage

120g (4¼oz) basmati rice
½ teaspoon ghee (see page 196) or olive oil
pinch of spice mix (see above)
½ spring cabbage, roughly chopped
12cm (4½in) stick of rhubarb, cut into batons, or the seeds of ¼ pomegranate
1 small leek, sliced into rounds
tamari soy sauce (optional)

Using a pestle and mortar, grind the ingredients for the spice mix to a fine powder.

Put the tofu in a small bowl and sprinkle in the spice mix, reserving a pinch for the cabbage. Use a spoon to gently turn the pieces of tofu in the powder to coat them. Then mix the tamari and sesame seeds into the tofu, cover and leave to marinate for at least 30 minutes.

While the tofu marinates, cook the rice according to the packet instructions. Drain the cooked rice and set aside.

Put the ghee or olive oil into a saucepan set over a medium–low heat, mix in the reserved spice mix and heat for a few moments to release some flavour. Add the cabbage, rhubarb (but not the pomegranate seeds, if substituting those for the rhubarb) and leek, plus a splash of water. Cover the pan with a lid and cook for 6–7 minutes until the vegetables are soft and cooked through, adding another splash of water, if necessary, to prevent sticking. When the vegetables are soft, stir in the cooked rice and a few dashes of tamari, if you like. (If you are using pomegranate seeds instead of rhubarb, add them at this point.)

While the cabbage is cooking, heat the ghee or oil in a frying pan over a medium–low heat and fry the marinated tofu for 6 minutes or so, until it has formed a slight crust on the edges.

Serve the rhubarb cabbage topped with the cooked tofu, sprinkled with chopped chives.

Tip

Keep your eyes open for artisan tofu makers – there is some exceptional-quality tofu out there to be had!

131

Butternut squash lasagne

Because it contains more vitamin A than any other vegetable, butternut squash is superb for supporting healthy skin and mucous membranes, and also helps you to see better in dim light. Adding nutmeg, ajwain seeds and cumin to the cheese sauce in this dish not only makes it delicious, but also helps the body to digest the squash better. Nutmeg is soothing to the nervous system. It imparts this quality to the dish, making it a comforting and satisfying meal.

Serves 2
Preparation time 20 minutes
Cooking time 1½ hours

3 large sheets of fresh pasta (see page 198) or use 6 dried lasagne sheets, cooked
handful of grated good-quality strong-flavoured cheese, such as Cheddar cheese

For the filling
1 tablespoon olive oil
1 small onion, finely chopped
2 garlic cloves, minced
700g (1lb 9oz) butternut squash, peeled and cut into small cubes
1 celery stick, finely chopped
½ teaspoon dried basil
½ teaspoon dried oregano
½ teaspoon paprika
½ teaspoon garlic powder
pinch of turmeric
150ml (¼ pint) boiling water, plus extra as necessary
½ head of broccoli, separated into florets
handful of peas
2 handfuls of chard or kale (use whole leaves)
unrefined salt and black pepper

For the cheese sauce
½ teaspoon ghee (see page 196)
1½ tablespoons spelt flour (or other flour of your choice)
250ml (9fl oz) rice milk or dairy milk
pinch of grated nutmeg
pinch of ground ajwain (carom) seeds
pinch of ground cumin
125g (4½oz) ricotta cheese, crumbled
unrefined salt and black pepper

Heat the oil in a large saucepan over a medium–low heat. Add the onion and fry gently for approximately 5 minutes, until translucent. Add the garlic and cook for a minute or so, then mix in the squash, celery, herbs and spices, and season with salt and pepper. Now stir in 100ml (3½fl oz) of the boiling water, reduce the heat to low, cover with a lid and simmer for 30 minutes, until the butternut squash is soft, adding extra water if the mixture begins to dry out.

Preheat the oven to 200°C/180°C fan (400°F), Gas Mark 6.

Stir the remaining boiling water into the pan along with the broccoli, and cook for a further 10 minutes until the broccoli is cooked. There should be a small amount of liquid left, giving the filling a sauce-like quality. Fold in the peas.

The chard or kale is used when layering the lasagne. If you are using kale, cook it while the broccoli is cooking. Put enough water to cover the kale into a saucepan, bring to a boil, then add the kale, reduce the heat to low and simmer for 5 minutes until soft. Drain and set aside.

You can also make the cheese sauce while the broccoli is cooking. Melt the ghee in a small saucepan, then add the flour, using a balloon whisk to blend it quickly with the ghee. Once combined, whisk continuously as you slowly pour in the rice or dairy milk, then continue to whisk for approximately 5 minutes, until the sauce is thick and smooth. Stir in the nutmeg, ajwain and cumin, season with salt and pepper, then stir in the ricotta and allow it to melt into the sauce. Take the pan off the heat and check the consistency of the sauce – it should be pourable. If it looks a little too thick, thin it out by whisking in just enough water to give it a pourable consistency.

Once the filling is cooked and the cheese sauce is done, assemble the lasagne in a 1 litre (1¾ pint) rectangular ovenproof dish. To create the first layer, pour one-quarter of the cheese sauce into the dish to cover the base. Cover this with 1 lasagne sheet, then spoon over half the vegetable mixture and spread it out evenly across the surface. Top with half the chard leaves or kale, then cover with one-third of the remaining cheese sauce. Now create the second layer. Lay down 1 lasagne sheet, then use the remaining vegetable mixture to cover the lasagne sheet in an even layer. Arrange the remaining greens on top of the filling and cover with

half the remaining cheese sauce. Cover with the final lasagne sheet, pour over the remaining cheese sauce and sprinkle over the grated cheese.

Bake for 40 minutes, until the top has browned nicely. Leave to cool for at least 5 minutes before serving, to allow the lasagne to firm up.

Tip
Pumpkin can be substituted for butternut squash in this recipe. If you are gluten free, either make your own gluten-free pasta or purchase gluten-free pasta sheets. If you are dairy free, omit the cheese from the sauce and sprinkle yeast flakes over the lasagne.

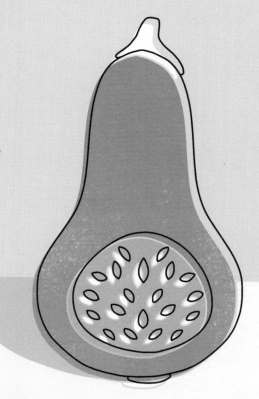

Packed lunch

According to Ayurveda, lunch should ideally be taken at
roughly the same time each day. It should be consumed while
seated, and your full attention and awareness should be given
to the consumption of your delicious, lovingly prepared meal.
That way, your digestive system will work optimally when
processing the meal. This leads to a reduction in bloating,
gas and other digestive disturbances later in the afternoon
and into the evening.

With a little planning ahead, a packed lunch can become
something exciting and delicious. In this section you will find
recipes for staple lunches that can replace sandwich-based
packed lunches. These recipes are designed to make the lunches
comparatively quick to make and easy to pack, but bear in mind
that all the recipes within the Lunch section can be cooked
the night before, reheated in the morning, transferred into a
food flask and taken to work for a nice, hot lunch. These are
more suited to the cooler months of the year while, conversely,
cold packed lunches are better in the warmer months.

Although you need to invest in some good-quality storage
containers and food flasks, regularly taking a packed lunch
to work with you will be much lighter on the pocket than a
reliance on purchased lunches. And having lunch in your bag
will encourage you not to skip this important meal if you
are too busy to leave your work station.

A note on sandwiches
Sandwiches are considered the root of many digestive
complaints, especially when consumed five days per week.
The fact that a sandwich is cold does not help, because all
the lovely phenols (the compounds that make food smell good
when it is heated) are not released to tickle your taste buds
and get the digestive juices flowing. And in the colder months,
the cold meal does not provide you with any inner warmth. But
the main reason why eating sandwiches for lunch every day is
a bad idea is because of the poor quality of the shop-bought
breads that are often used to make them. Those breads, often
made with highly processed ingredients combined with quick-

acting yeast, are low in nutritional value, providing limited fuel for the afternoon, which often leads to a mid-afternoon slump in energy — and then to food cravings.

Remember that the sense of smell is vital when it comes to initiating good digestion. Also, all the taste receptors need to be stimulated through a range of six tastes; sweet, sour, salty, bitter, pungent and astringent. Because it is difficult to stimulate the gustatory system properly with a sandwich, digestion is not sparked into full process, leading to excessive weight, especially around the waistline, and sluggish energy levels. It is, of course, possible to include all of the tastes within one sandwich. For instance, some gourmet sandwiches include pickles and spices, which can bridge the taste gaps. They are also often made with bread such as sourdough, soda bread or rye, which are all much better for the digestive system. So, if you are dedicated to sandwiches in the warmer months, all these challenges can be overcome — especially if you make your own bread using wholesome ingredients.

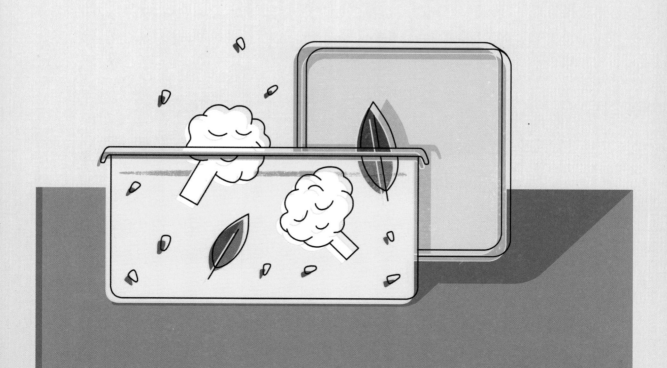

Courgette, puy lentil and rosemary scoffins _____

The scoffin lies somewhere between a muffin and a scone, and it provides the perfect portable lunch. The liberal addition of olive oil helps to counterbalance the astringent and drying nature of lentils. The rosemary and thyme give the scoffins a delicious flavour, and also help to enhance digestive functioning and prevent the production of excessive gas due to lentil consumption.

Makes 8 scoffins
Preparation time 10 minutes, plus soaking and cooling
Cooking time 35 minutes

150g (5½oz) spelt flour
2 teaspoons baking powder
2 tablespoons olive oil
80ml (2¾fl oz) water
50g (1¾oz) Puy or green lentils, soaked for
   at least 4 hours, then cooked until soft
½ courgette, grated
1 teaspoon chopped fresh rosemary
1 teaspoon chopped fresh thyme
pinch of paprika
unrefined salt and black pepper

Preheat the oven to 200°C/180°C fan (400°F), Gas Mark 6. Line a muffin tin with 8 paper muffin cases.

Put all the ingredients into a bowl and mix well to form a lovely fluffy mixture.

Divide the mixture between the prepared muffin cases (or spoon it straight into a greased and floured muffin tin). Bake for 35 minutes, until light brown on the top and a skewer inserted into the centre of a scoffin comes out clean. Leave to cool before packing for lunch or putting into an airtight container for another day.

Tips
• A scoffin is delicious served with a salad and hummus in the warmer months, and makes a great accompaniment to soups and vegetable dishes in the colder months of the year. Leftovers from many of the dishes in the Dinner section of this book can be reheated in the morning and packed into a flask, to be enjoyed with a scoffin at lunchtime.

• If you wish to use tinned lentils, use roughly half a 400g (14oz) can, drained and rinsed.

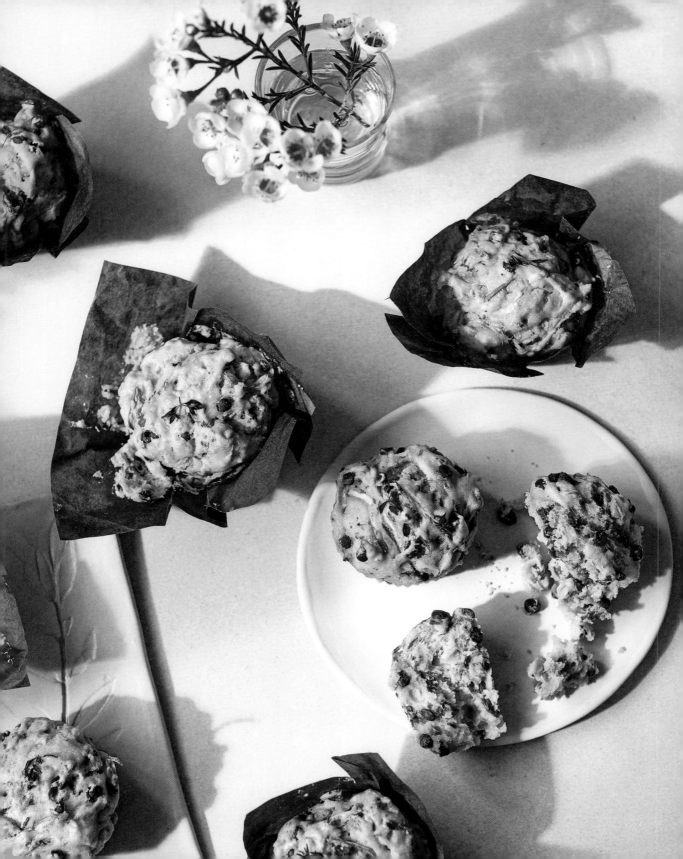

Sweet potato and pea tortilla

Eggs are a good source of nourishment, supportive to the reproductive system and are very grounding. Having said that, some people find they have a slightly binding action in the intestines and can be somewhat heavy for digestion. Adding rosemary, which promotes good digestion, helps to mitigate this.

Serves 2
Preparation time 5 minutes
Cooking time 15–20 minutes

1 sweet potato, peeled and diced
1 small leek, sliced
4 free-range eggs
1 tablespoon chopped dried seaweed
  (optional)
1 teaspoon chopped fresh rosemary
¼ teaspoon smoked paprika
¼ teaspoon ghee (see page 196)
  or ½ teaspoon olive oil
handful of frozen peas
unrefined salt and black pepper

Put the sweet potato and leek into a medium-sized deep ovenproof frying pan. Add just enough water to cover the veg, cover the frying pan with a lid and simmer gently over a medium heat for approximately 10 minutes, until the vegetables are soft – by this point, the water should have evaporated.

Meanwhile, put the eggs, seaweed (if using), rosemary and smoked paprika into a measuring jug, season with salt and pepper, then beat with a fork to combine the ingredients.

Preheat your grill.

When the sweet potato is cooked, add the ghee and peas to the frying pan and fry all the vegetables together gently for 1 minute. Then pour the egg mixture over the top and cover the pan with a lid. Reduce the heat to medium–low and cook for around 3 minutes, until the mixture has set on the underside. Remove the lid, transfer the pan to the grill and cook for 2–3 minutes, to finish cooking the egg on the top.

Transfer the tortilla to a chopping board and leave to cool completely, then cut it into sections and pack in an airtight container.

Tip
You can make this tortilla the night before. It keeps well if refrigerated overnight.

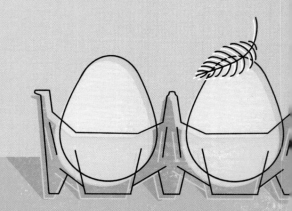

Heating butternut squash and noodle salad _____

This lunch dish is highly suited to autumn and winter, when mucus is beginning to increase in the body and the air is damp. Through the use of chilli, ginger and sage, it helps to keep the respiratory tract clear by drawing out excess secretions. The bright and colourful butternut squash, being full of vitamins and minerals, acts as a tonic – and it also gives you a burst of sunshine on a cold and miserable day! If you suffer from inflammatory skin conditions or generally from excess heat, omit the chilli.

Serves 2
Preparation time 10 minutes
Cooking time 10 minutes

1 teaspoon sunflower oil
1cm (½in) piece of fresh root ginger, peeled and finely chopped
½ small red chilli, deseeded and finely diced
4 spring onions, chopped
150g (5½oz) butternut squash, peeled and cut into thin batons
2 tablespoons water
handful of kale or spring greens, shredded
5 sage leaves, chopped
½ teaspoon chopped dried seaweed salad
handful of cooked chestnuts (or use pistachio nuts), chopped
tamari soy sauce
200g (7oz) buckwheat noodles, cooked according to the packet instructions

Heat the oil in a large wok or frying pan over a medium heat, then add the ginger and chilli and fry for 1–2 minutes to release their aromas. Stir in the spring onion and butternut squash, add the measured water, cover the pan with a lid and cook for 3–4 minutes. The butternut squash should just be beginning to soften – when you insert a knife, they will have a bit of give, but in essence are still firm.

Stir the kale or spring greens, chopped sage, seaweed and chestnuts into the pan, then cover the pan with a lid and cook for a further 4 minutes, until the kale or greens are cooked.

To finish, shake a liberal amount of tamari over the vegetables, mix it in, then toss in the cooked noodles.

Pack the mixture into a food flask while hot, or allow it to cool completely, then pack in an airtight container.

Tip
In the spring, make this with sprouting broccoli, asparagus, wild garlic and walnuts. During the summer months, make this with courgettes and cashew nuts. Omit the chili and sage, and add coriander or mint leaves instead.

Roasted cauliflower and kale quinoa pot _____

Cauliflower and kale are brassicas and are available throughout the winter and into spring. They are highly nutritious and are considered to be prebiotics, encouraging good gut bacteria to thrive due to the glucosinolates they contain, which are broken down by gut bacteria to release desirable health-promoting and disease-fighting compounds. These compounds have been shown to inhibit the growth of cancer. They also contain sulphur, however, and have a tendency to produce excess gas through the digestion process. Adding cumin gives the vegetable a lovely flavour and also prevents excess gas production.

Serves 1
Preparation time 5 minutes
Cooking time 15–20 minutes

For the cauliflower
½ cauliflower, broken into florets
2 large kale leaves, finely chopped
  (trim and discard the central stalks)
1 leek, roughly chopped
1 teaspoon cumin seeds
1 teaspoon olive oil or ½ teaspoon ghee
  (see page 196)
1 teaspoon ground cashew nuts
unrefined salt and black pepper

For the quinoa
60g (2¼oz) quinoa
1 tablespoon olive oil
unrefined salt and black pepper

For the topping
1 teaspoon sunflower seeds
small slice of soft goats' cheese
small squeeze of lemon juice

Preheat the oven to 200°C/180°C fan (400°F), Gas Mark 6.

Bring some water to a boil in a steamer pan, put the cauliflower, kale and leek into the steamer basket and steam for 6–8 minutes, until the cauliflower is just tender.

Transfer the lightly steamed vegetables to a baking dish, sprinkle over the cumin seeds, drizzle with oil or ghee, season with salt and pepper, then toss the vegetables to coat in the oil. Bake for 7–10 minutes, until the cauliflower has crisped and browned on the edges a little. Sprinkle over the cashew nuts and return the dish to the oven for 1 minute to toast the nuts.

While the vegetables are cooking, cook the quinoa according to the packet instructions. It is ready when the little 'tails' uncurl and the grains are soft but still retain some bite. Drain the cooked quinoa, transfer it to a large bowl, then drizzle liberally with olive oil and season with salt and pepper.

When the vegetables are cooked, mix them into the prepared quinoa. Transfer the hot mixture to a storage flask and top with sunflower seeds and goats' cheese and squeeze over some lemon juice. Alternatively, allow the mixture to cool, then pack it into an airtight container.

Tip
This recipe uses a winter selection of vegetables, which can be substituted with sweet peppers, fennel and courgette in the summer and can be prepared in a similar way, just shortening the roasting time to 5 minutes.

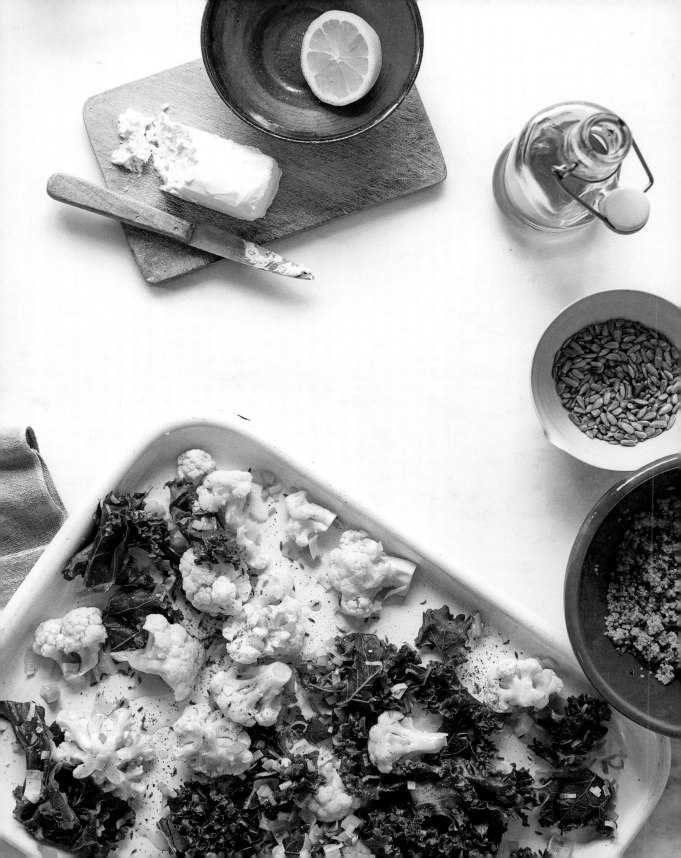

Warm-weather three-minute couscous

According to Ayurveda, fresh tomatoes should be enjoyed in season and when very ripe. The skins, which are harder to digest, are discarded. Fennel is both sweet and sour and is very aromatic in its raw form. Its volatile oil compounds stimulate the digestion system through both aroma and taste, making it easy to digest uncooked. It has a natural sweetness that is balancing for the body in warm weather. Coriander and fennel are cooling and counterbalance any heat from the tomatoes.

Serves 1
Preparation time 5 minutes, plus cooling

For the couscous
100g (3½oz) couscous
160ml (5½fl oz) boiling water
2 tablespoons olive oil
1 tablespoon chopped fresh coriander
1 large ripe tomato
pinch of ground cumin
1 fennel bulb, thinly sliced
handful of mixed lettuce leaves
1 tablespoon pumpkin seeds
1 tablespoon crushed walnuts
1 tablespoon shaved Parmesan cheese or
   1 tablespoon Cumin Labneh (see page 201)
unrefined salt and black pepper

Put the couscous into a bowl and pour over the measured boiling water. Cover the bowl with a plate and leave to stand for 2 minutes, then use a fork to fluff up the couscous. If, by this time, the couscous has absorbed all the water, it is ready. If not, re-cover with the plate and leave to stand for another minute or so before checking and fluffing again. When the couscous is ready, season with salt and pepper to taste, drizzle over the olive oil, then mix in the chopped coriander. Leave to cool.

Meanwhile, immerse the tomato in some boiling water and leave to stand for a few minutes until its skin cracks. Then carefully remove the tomato from the water using a slotted spoon and slip its skin off. Discard the skin and seeds and dice the tomato flesh. Put the tomato into a bowl, sprinkle over the cumin, then mix in the fennel, lettuce, pumpkin seeds and crushed walnuts.

When ready to pack, put the couscous into an airtight container and top with the tomato mixture. Finally, top with the shaved Parmesan or cumin labneh and seal.

Tip
The raw ingredients included in this lunch dish make it suitable for warm weather. (Generally, it is best to enjoy cooked food when it is cold outside.) The calorific content of this meal is low, which is suited to hot-weather days when the body's calorific requirements are naturally low and, therefore, digestive capacity is lower.

Refuelling rice and red lentil balls _____

The combination of rice and red lentils in these power balls provides a very easily digestible source of protein, making them nourishing and sustaining. You can get creative with the coatings for these balls, decorating them in all sorts of ways, making them a true delight for the senses. I have suggested three types of coatings, and you can mix these in with the ingredients for the balls instead, if you do not have the inclination to coat them. To vary the flavours further, add a pinch of the appropriate seasonal spice mix (see pages 55, 58, 62 and 65). Alternatively, add a dash of whatever spices take your fancy today. Let your sense of smell be your guide!

Serves 2
Preparation time 10 minutes, plus soaking and cooling
Cooking time 20 minutes

1 leek, diced
1 celery stick, diced
100g (3½oz) basmati rice
60g (2¼oz) red lentils, soaked for at least
  4 hours
400ml (14fl oz) hot vegetable stock
½ teaspoon dried basil
½ teaspoon olive oil or ghee (see page 196)
pinch of seasonal spice mix (optional, see
  pages 55, 58, 62 and 65)
tamari soy sauce
handful of spinach leaves or nori seaweed
  or 1 tablespoon sesame seeds
unrefined salt and black pepper

Place the leek, celery, rice, lentils and stock in a saucepan, add the basil and oil or ghee, and season with salt and pepper. If you are adding one of the seasonal spice mixes, add a pinch of that too. Simmer gently over a medium–low heat for as long as directed by the cooking instructions on the rice packet, so that the lentils have turned yellow and are softish, and the rice is cooked. This will take approximately 20 minutes, by which time, all the water should have been absorbed by the rice, but if there is any water left in the pan, drain it away carefully. Allow the mixture to cool slightly, then add a couple of dashes of tamari to taste.

Cook the spinach (if using) while the rice mixture is cooking. Set a medium saucepan over a low heat and pour in just enough boiling water to cover the base. Put a steamer basket on top of the saucepan, add the spinach leaves and cook gently for 2 minutes, until the leaves have wilted. Set aside.

Spread the rice and lentils mixture across a large dinner plate and leave to cool and firm up for 5–10 minutes. Then scoop out 1 tablespoon of the rice mixture and, with wet hands, gently compress it into a ball between your palms, then place into an airtight container or food flask. Continue in this way until you have around 24 balls, then place the spinach on the side and seal. Alternatively, wrap each ball in spinach leaves or seaweed, or roll in sesame seeds, before packing.

Tip
For a warm lunch in the cold months, transfer the rice and lentil mixture to a food flask as soon as it's cooked, folding in the cooked spinach, nori or sesame seeds, and seal immediately to keep the heat in.

143

Protein power pot

When you open your flask at lunchtime, the wonderful aroma of fresh herbs will be immediately released, helping to get the digestive juices flowing. Quinoa and red lentils together provide an easily digestible source of protein to keep you going all afternoon. Use seasonal herbs to benefit from their health properties.

Serves 1
Preparation time 5 minutes, plus soaking
Cooking time 20–22 minutes

60g (2¼oz) quinoa
60g (2¼oz) red lentils, soaked for at least
   4 hours
1 shallot, diced
¼ courgette, diced
350ml (12fl oz) boiling water
¼ teaspoon vegetable bouillon powder
1cm (½in) piece of fresh root ginger, peeled
   and finely chopped
drizzle of olive oil or ½ teaspoon ghee
   (see page 196)
3 broccoli florets
1½ tablespoons chopped seasonal fresh
   green herbs (mint works particularly well)
unrefined salt and black pepper

To garnish
splash of tamari soy sauce
1 teaspoon pumpkin seeds

Place all the ingredients, except the broccoli and herbs, into a saucepan and simmer over a medium–low heat for 20 minutes, adding more water to the pan if the mixture looks as though it is drying out.

Once 12 minutes of the cooking time have elapsed, lightly steam the broccoli in a steamer pan.

When the cooking time for the quinoa and lentils mixture has elapsed, the water should have been absorbed and both the quinoa and lentils should be soft and moist. Mix in the steamed broccoli and chopped herbs.

To pack a warm lunch in the winter months, spoon the mixture into a food flask at this point. Splash over tamari to taste, top with the pumpkin seeds and seal.

In the summer months, allow the mixture to cool, transfer to an airtight container and store at room temperature until lunchtime.

Tip
In springtime, add some young nettles leaves or wild garlic during the cooking process. In summer, fold in some rocket leaves, fresh mint or parsley when you mix in the chopped herbs. In the winter, add some sage during the cooking process.

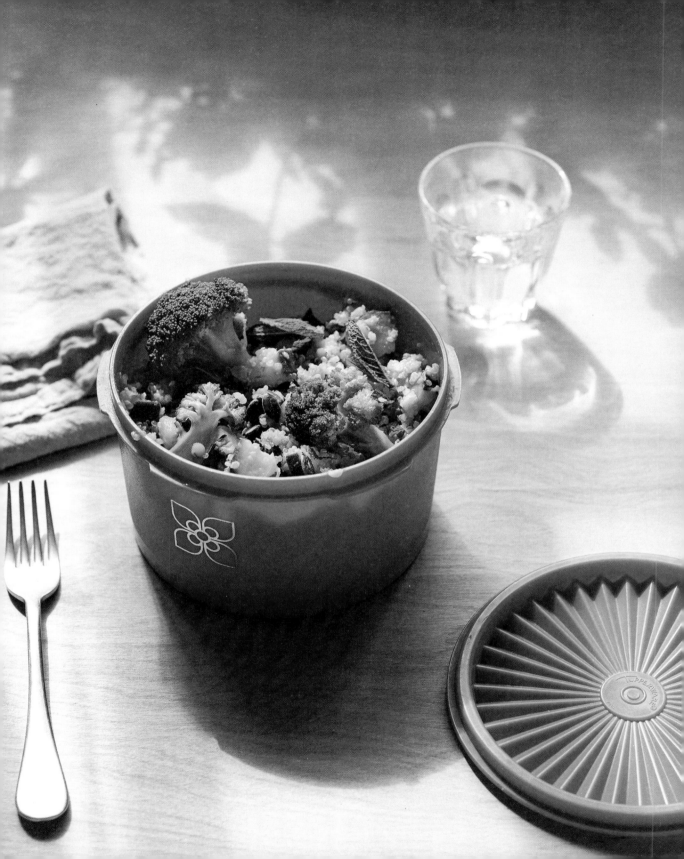

Easy homemade wraps

This recipe suggests three variations for the filling, including an option using goats' cheese – one of the few dairy cheeses that most people can digest well. As with all cheeses, it can still produce excess mucus, but this is overcome by combining it with cumin seeds and peppers. You can, of course, devise fillings of your own for the delicious flatbreads. By including rosemary in them, the heavy properties of the flour are counterbalanced, promoting better digestion of the gluten. You can substitute gluten-free flour if required; this will just require less kneading.

Serves 2
Preparation time 15 minutes, plus cooling
Cooking time 20 minutes

For the pepper filling
1 teaspoon olive oil
1 red pepper, cored, deseeded and
   sliced lengthways
2 spring onions or 1 red onion, chopped
pinch of ground cumin
4 tablespoons water
handful of spinach

For the flatbreads
150g (5½oz) white spelt flour, plus extra
   for dusting
1 teaspoon baking powder
1 teaspoon chopped rosemary
pinch of unrefined salt
2 tablespoons olive oil
80ml (2¾fl oz) water

Additional fillings
6 small slices of goats' cheese, or
   4 tablespoons Cumin Labneh (see page
   201) or Sprouted Chickpea Hummus
   (see page 200)
2 tablespoons lightly crushed walnuts

Preheat the oven to 200°C/180°C fan (400°F), Gas Mark 6.

To make the pepper filling, heat the oil in a frying pan over a low heat. Add the pepper, onion and cumin and gently fry for 2 minutes, then add the measured water, cover the pan with a lid and simmer for approximately 15 minutes, until the peppers are soft.

Meanwhile, make the flatbreads. Place the flour, baking powder, rosemary and salt in a large bowl and mix thoroughly. Make a well in the centre of the mixture and pour the oil and measured water into it. Using a wooden spoon, stir the mixture until it combines in a ball. Dust your work top with a little flour, then knead the dough for 5–10 minutes, until smooth and pliable. Cover the dough with a clean, damp cloth and leave it to rest on the countertop for 5 minutes, then cut it into 6 equal segments.

By now the peppers should be soft, so toss in the spinach, turn off the heat and leave the lid on the frying pan. If you are packing your lunch during the colder months, as soon as the spinach has wilted, transfer the pepper mixture to a food flask. In the warm months, allow the mixture to cool completely, then transfer to an airtight container.

Return to the flatbreads. Using a rolling pin, roll each of the dough segments into thin circles with a diameter of 18cm (7in). Place these on baking sheets, transfer to the oven and bake for 2–3 minutes, until cooked. Stack the cooked flatbreads, straight out of the oven, on a plate and place another upturned plate on top so that the breads are completely enclosed – this keeps them pliable. Store the flatbreads in this way until cooled, then roll them into cylinders and place in an airtight container.

To complete packing your lunch, put some sliced goats' cheese, cumin labneh or homemade hummus and the walnuts into an airtight storage container. Wrap up the flatbread separately. Add the packed peppers to the lunch bag. At lunchtime, roll up the wraps and enjoy.

Tips

- If you are making up the components of this packed lunch the night before, store the pepper mixture in an airtight container in the refrigerator overnight. To keep the flatbreads pliable, leave them stacked between the plates or store them in a bag at room temperature.

- Use your leftovers from the day before as wrap fillings. These flatbreads work well with any vegetables, lentils or beans. It is a good idea to cook larger portions of your meals with this in mind.

- During the spring and summer months, substitute fresh watercress or pea shoots for spinach in the pepper filling. These leaves do not need to be cooked – simply stir them into the pepper mixture at the end of cooking.

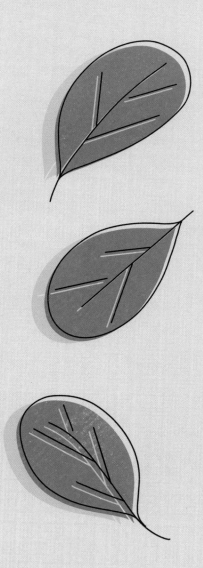

Dinner

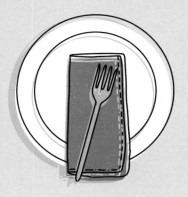

Ideally, your supper should be the lightest meal of the day in order to ensure good-quality sleep. The body rests and rejuvenates overnight better if it is not processing a heavy meal. Furthermore, heavy meals consumed later at night tend not to be digested properly, resulting in feelings of sluggishness, lethargy and low appetite in the morning. If you are someone who has a low appetite early in the day, this might be because you are eating too much too late in the evenings.

Keeping evening meals light and warm allows them to be well digested. When food is cooked, the cellulose structures are broken down, so less effort is required on the part of the digestive system to absorb the nutrients.

If your work routine dictates that your evening meal must be the largest, try to eat it as early as possible in the evening.

Pre-dinner exercise

Once your dinner is cooking, often there is a little nugget
of spare time while you wait for it to finish. Take advantage
of that window to perform this brief pre-dinner exercise,
which helps you release the day's tension from your neck
and upper back.

Preparation Stand with your feet hip-width apart, with a
soft bend in the knees. Lift your toes, stretch and spread
them out. Now as you return them to the floor, claw at it
with the tips of your toes and engage the arches of your feet.
Now relax the toes. Feel yourself lifting up through your
legs. Lift your chest slightly and drop your shoulders. Take
a couple of smooth, long breaths. Join your hands together in
prayer position in front of your chest. Take a full complete
breath in, feeling your ribcage expanding.

Exercise sequence As you exhale, slowly lower your chin to your
chest. Inhale as you return your head to centre. Exhale and
look up towards the ceiling. Inhale and return your head to
centre. Exhale and turn your head to look to your right. Inhale
and return your head to centre. Exhale and turn you head to
look to your left. Inhale and return your head to centre.

Nourishing spiced pumpkin soup

Pumpkin is packed with B vitamins, vitamins A and C, and minerals, particularly potassium. It is perfect for consumption in the autumn, as it combats the drying properties of the autumnal winds and any accumulation of heat in the body following a long summer. The spices combined with the pumpkin in this dish complement its flavour well and help to make the properties of the pumpkin more bioavailable.

Serves 1
Preparation time 7 minutes
Cooking time 22 minutes

1 teaspoon olive oil or ghee (see page 196)
pinch of black pepper
pinch of ground coriander
pinch of ground cumin
1cm (½in) piece of fresh root ginger, peeled
   and roughly chopped
1 celery stick, chopped
1 leek, chopped
350g (12oz) pumpkin, peeled and roughly
   chopped
450ml (16fl oz) hot vegetable stock
1 tablespoon pumpkin seeds, for sprinkling

Heat the oil or ghee in a large saucepan over a low heat. Add the spices and ginger and fry for 1–2 minutes, until the spices release their aromas, then stir in the celery, leek, pumpkin and vegetable stock. Simmer for 20 minutes, until the pumpkin is soft.

Take the pan off the heat and allow the mixture to cool slightly, then blitz with a handheld blender or transfer to a blender and blend until smooth. Alternatively, carefully mash the soup by hand with a potato masher.

Transfer to a bowl, top with the pumpkin seeds and serve immediately.

Tips
- Eat this soup once daily for a few days during the change of season from summer to autumn, to help balance the digestive system and, thus, the body.

- Soda Bread (see page 110) or a good-quality sourdough bread make a delicious accompaniment to this soup.

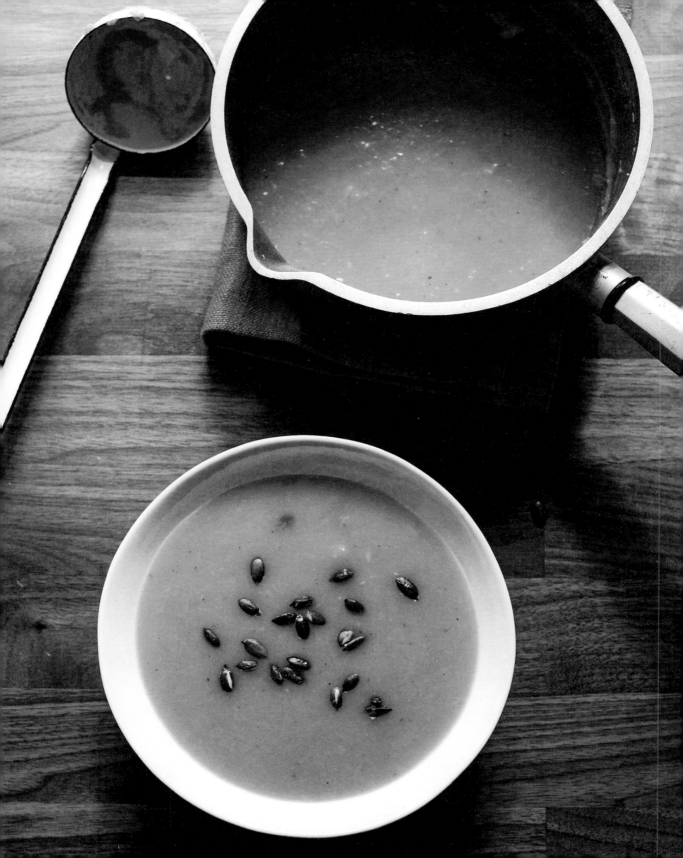

Digestion-enhancing pak choi and noodle broth _____

The combination of fresh ginger, star anise and lemon grass in this broth gently lifts the digestive capacity without stimulating excessive heat or acidity. Pak choi is a member of the brassica family and is very high in antioxidants and vitamin C. For this reason, it is better to cook it for the minimum amount of time possible, to retain its health-promoting properties. Lemon grass is both pungent and bitter. It is both a pain reliever and anti-inflammatory. It can be helpful in arthritis, for fevers, coughs and colds, and it supports the digestive system.

Serves 1
Preparation time 7 minutes
Cooking time 12–15 minutes

1 lemon grass stalk, peeled and
   roughly chopped
2cm (¾in) piece of fresh root ginger, peeled
   and roughly chopped
1 small red onion, roughly chopped
1 small garlic clove, roughly chopped
½ teaspoon ghee (see page 196)
400ml (14fl oz) hot vegetable or chicken stock
1 teaspoon tamari soy sauce, plus a few
   dashes extra
1 star anise
1 celery stick, cut into thin strips
1 head of pak choi, roughly chopped
1 portion of udon, rice or buckwheat noodles
1 tablespoon cashew nuts
¼ teaspoon lime juice
few grinds of black pepper
1 teaspoon sesame seeds, to garnish

Place the lemon grass, ginger, red onion and garlic into a spice grinder and grind to a paste. (Alternatively, grind them to a paste using a pestle and mortar.)

Heat the ghee in a medium saucepan over a medium–low heat. Add the paste and heat gently for 2–3 minutes its aromas to be released, stirring continuously. Stir in the stock, tamari and star anise and simmer gently for 5 minutes, then mix in the celery and pak choi and season with pepper. Continue to cook for a further 5 minutes, until the celery and pak choi are cooked.

In the meantime, cook the noodles according to the packet instructions.

While the noodles and broth are cooking, place the cashew nuts in a saucepan over medium heat, stir in a few dashes of tamari and heat the nuts gently for 1 minute.

When the celery and pak choi are cooked, stir the lime juice into the pan, followed by the cooked noodles and cashew nuts.

Serve immediately in a wide bowl, with sesame seeds sprinkled on top.

Tip
Try growing your own lemon grass on your kitchen windowsill. This is such a fun and easy thing to do. Buy a fresh lemon grass stalk, immerse the lower third of it in some water in a jar and leave it on a windowsill. After around a week, shoots should appear from its base. Once they are 1–2cm (½–¾in) in length, plant the stalk in compost in a deep pot. Keep it on a windowsill and water it regularly. Over time, those shoots will turn into new plants that will spring up.

Blood-boosting beetroot soup

Iron-rich beetroot is very sweet. Both the sage and radishes in this dish balance its sweet taste and help to ensure it is properly digested, so that all its wonderful iron can be absorbed by the body. Radish is a fabulous vegetable for kindling the digestive fire. If you find your digestive system is sluggish, you may choose to add more radishes to the dish, or even some horseradish.

Serves 2
Preparation time 10 minutes
Cooking time 50 minutes

1 red onion, diced
2 large beetroot, chopped
up to 6 radishes (as per your desired
  pungency), roughly chopped
700ml (1¼ pints) water
2 teaspoons vegetable bouillon powder
4 sage leaves
splash of olive oil
black pepper

Place all the ingredients into a saucepan over a medium–high heat and bring to a boil. Reduce the heat to medium–low and simmer for 45 minutes, until the beetroot is soft.

Take the pan off the heat. Pass the soup through a sieve, collecting the stock in a measuring jug. Transfer the contents of the sieve to a pot or large jug that is suitable for blending and add 150ml (¼ pint) of the collected stock. (Retain any leftover stock to thin the soup, if required, or to add to other sauces.) Allow the mixture to cool a little, then blitz with a handheld blender. Return the soup to the saucepan to reheat for 1–2 minutes, then serve.

Tips

- This soup goes well with the Scoffins on page 136 in a packed lunch.

- If radishes are unavailable, substitute a 1cm (½in) piece of fresh root ginger, roughly chopped.

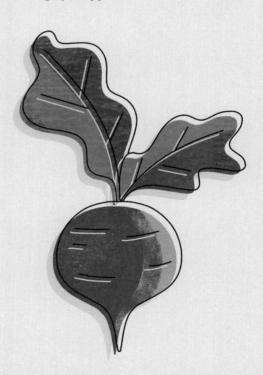

Slow-cooked barley and mung beans _____

Barley is full of fibre and protein. It promotes fat metabolism and aids the digestive system. Mung beans add even more protein to the pot. The bay and thyme further support the digestive system and help to negate any tendency of the barley and beans to cause bloating or gas.

Serves 2
Preparation time 5 minutes
Cooking time 8–10 hours

75g (2¾oz) pearl barley
100g (3½oz) mung beans
1 carrot, peeled and chopped
1 parsnip, diced
1 onion, thinly sliced
2 garlic cloves, with skin left on
2 bay leaves
4 sprigs of fresh thyme
pinch of coarsely ground black pepper
850ml (1½ pints) water
2 teaspoons vegetable bouillon powder
1 teaspoon olive oil

To garnish
handful of seasonal greens, such as
   dandelion, spinach or pea shoots,
   roughly chopped
squeeze of lemon juice

Place all the ingredients in a slow cooker in the order listed. Put the lid on the pot and cook on the lowest setting for 8 hours. When cooked, most, if not all of the stock will have been absorbed by the barley.

When you are ready to serve, stir in some additional boiling water if it looks and tastes a little too dry, then mix in the chopped greens and reheat to warm and moisten. Add a squeeze of lemon to serve.

Tips
- The advantage of a slow cooker is you can put it on in the morning and your meal is ready in the evening. If you do not have one, however, you can soak the beans and barley overnight for extra digestive comfort, then cook this dish in the oven in a casserole pot. Cook at 170°C/150°C fan (340°F), Gas Mark 3½ for 2–3 hours.

- In the summer, substitute beetroot for the parsnip. You can, in fact, use any seasonal root vegetable.

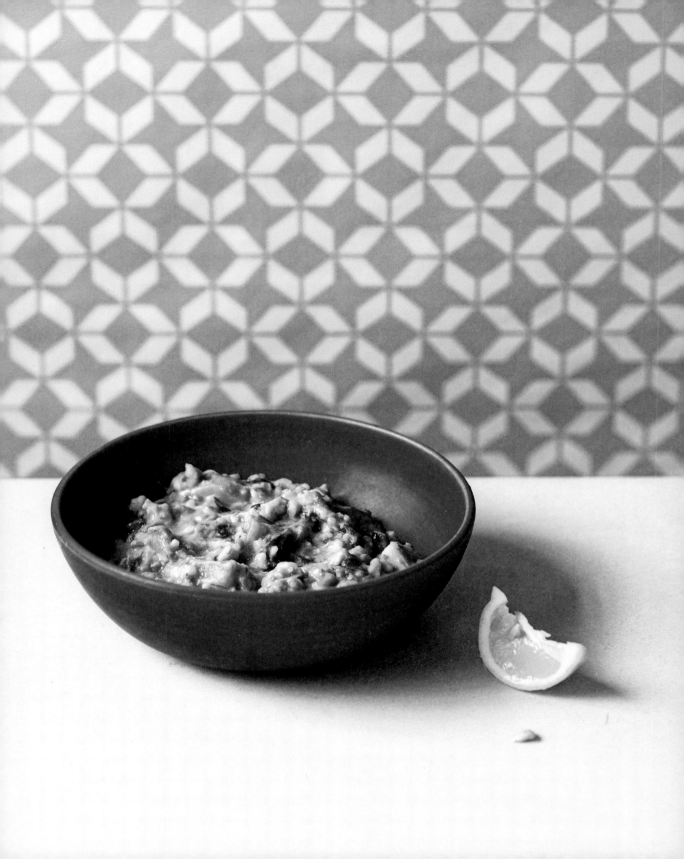

Quick-cook red lentil mini-stew _____

Red lentils are easier to digest than other pulses, as they have a less fibrous husk and, therefore, produce less gas. They make a great base ingredient for a stew and contain high amounts of folate, which is needed for healthy cell production and is important during pregnancy. Red lentils are sweet in taste and can be drying, so it helps to combine them with a little fat in combination with nourishing grains like bulgur wheat or rice. Using asafoetida in cooking helps to prevent the formation of gas from beans or pulses.

Serves 2
Preparation time 5 minutes, plus soaking
Cooking time 15 minutes

50g (1¾oz) dried red lentils, soaked for
    at least 4 hours
50g (1¾oz) bulgur wheat, rice or quinoa
1 leek, chopped
½ teaspoon chopped fresh root ginger
400ml (14fl oz) water
½ teaspoon vegetable bouillon powder
small pinch of turmeric
tiny pinch of asafoetida
1 teaspoon chopped fresh sage, thyme
    or parsley
drizzle of olive oil or ¼ teaspoon ghee
    (see page 196)
handful of purple sprouting broccoli,
    roughly chopped
unrefined salt and black pepper

To garnish
¼ lemon
1 tablespoon cashew nuts, lightly crushed
seasonal fresh green herbs, roughly
    chopped or torn

Place all the ingredients, except the broccoli, in a saucepan and bring to a boil over a high heat. Then reduce the heat to medium–low and simmer, stirring occasionally, for 15 minutes, until the bulgur wheat (or rice or quinoa) and lentils are cooked (the lentils will turn yellow and soft).

Once 10 minutes of the cooking time has elapsed, steam the broccoli in a steamer pan for 5 minutes, until cooked and still bright purple.

When the cooking time for the lentils and bulgur wheat (or rice or quinoa) has elapsed, the mixture should have a wet, but not soup-like, consistency – you may need to add a little extra water towards the end of cooking. Add a squeeze of lemon juice, the broccoli and the cashew nuts, season with salt and pepper to taste, garnish with fresh green herbs and serve immediately.

Tips
- This recipe offers a simpler alternative to traditional Cleansing Kitchari (see page 157). For seasonal variations, try adding different vegetables. For example, add a handful of both sweet potato and cavolo nero in the autumn and winter. You can also add a pinch of seasonal spice mix (see pages 55, 58, 62 and 65) with 4 tablespoons tomato passata when you feel like something a bit richer.

- In Ayurveda, it is recommended that red lentils are consumed if you are suffering from a fever. So, if you are unwell with a fever, remove the grain from this recipe to produce more of a soup, and eat a bowlful for lunch and dinner.

Cleansing kitchari _____

Kitchari is considered to be the sole recipe required for a healthy body. The combination of fat, mung beans, rice, vegetables and spices means that all dietary requirements are met, so feel free to enjoy it several times per week. Kitchari can additionally be consumed two to three times per day for several days in a row as a cleansing process. It kindles the digestive fire and clears much metabolic waste from the body, leaving you feeling light and full of energy. Mung beans are sweet and cold in potency and very slightly drying, so combining them with spices and some fat counterbalances these innate properties.

Serves 2
Preparation time 5 minutes, plus soaking
Cooking time 25–30 minutes

1 teaspoon ghee (see page 196)
1 teaspoon chopped fresh root ginger
½ teaspoon ground cumin
¼ teaspoon turmeric
½ teaspoon ground coriander seeds
tiny pinch of asafoetida
100g (3½oz) basmati rice
100g (3½oz) mung beans, soaked for
 at least 4 hours
600ml (20fl oz) water
2 bay leaves
unrefined salt and black pepper

To garnish
¼ lemon
1 tablespoon chopped fresh herbs,
 such as coriander or flat leaf parsley

Heat the ghee in a large saucepan over a medium–low heat, then add the spices and mix well. Stir in the remaining ingredients and bring the mixture to a boil, then reduce the heat to medium–low and simmer for 20–30 minutes, or as directed on on the rice packet. There should be very little water left at the end of the cooking process. Keep an eye on the kitchari during cooking, as you may need to add a little extra water if it is drying out too much.

To serve, squeeze some lemon juice onto the kitchari and sprinkle over the freshly chopped herbs.

Tip
- Add fresh herbs according to the season when you are cooking kitchari – try thyme in the spring, coriander in the summer, and oregano and basil from windowsill pots in the autumn and winter.

- Add fresh seasonal vegetables to the mix when you are not using the recipe as part of the Seasonal Reset Ritual on page 52.

Light-to-digest spelt flour pizza _____

Traditionally, fast-action yeast is used to leaven pizza dough, but I've avoided it in this recipe as it can cause digestive issues for some. If you happen to make your own sourdough bread, you can use your starter with this recipe (see tip) – yeast from a good sourdough starter promotes excellent assimilation of the flour. The basil and olive oil help to counterbalance the inflammatory effect that tomatoes have on some people. Removing the tomato skins and seeds tends to minimize their inflammatory potential too.

Serves 2
Preparation time 20 minutes
Cooking time 10–12 minutes

For the pizza dough
150g (5½oz) spelt flour, plus extra for dusting
1 teaspoon cream of tartar or baking powder
¼ teaspoon bicarbonate of soda
1 tablespoon olive oil
80ml (2¾fl oz) water
pinch of unrefined salt

For the tomato sauce
1 fresh ripe tomato
1 teaspoon olive oil
1½ teaspoons dried basil
tiny pinch of turmeric
unrefined salt and black pepper

For the topping
1 small beetroot, freshly cooked and sliced
75g (2¾oz) goats' cheese or other soft
  white cheese, such as ricotta cheese

Preheat the oven to 220°C/200°C fan (425°F), Gas Mark 7.

Put all the pizza dough ingredients into a large bowl and combine with your hands to form a dough. Separate the dough into 4 equal balls (or 2 larger balls, if you prefer). Dust your work top with flour, then roll out each portion to form a thin pizza base that is either round or slightly oval in shape. Transfer the dough bases to a baking sheet.

Put the tomato sauce ingredients into the jug of a blender and liquidize the mixture. Liberally spoon the sauce onto the pizzas. Finish by topping the pizzas with the sliced beetroot and cheese.

Bake for approximately 6 minutes, then open the oven door and, using a fish slice, gently slide the pizzas off the baking sheets directly onto the oven racks. Cook for a further 4 minutes, until the top of the pizzas turn golden brown and the undersides are firm.

Transfer the cooked pizzas to a chopping board, slice and enjoy.

Tips
* This recipe can be adapted to make perfect mini pizzas to serve as an hors d'oeuvres at a party. Divide the dough into 16 balls and roll out mini pizza bases, then top and cook as directed.

* To make the pizza base with a sourdough starter, omit the cream of tartar and bicarbonate of soda. Add 85g (3oz) sourdough starter that has been activated overnight. Combine it with the remaining dough ingredients and leave to prove for 4 hours before rolling out to cook.

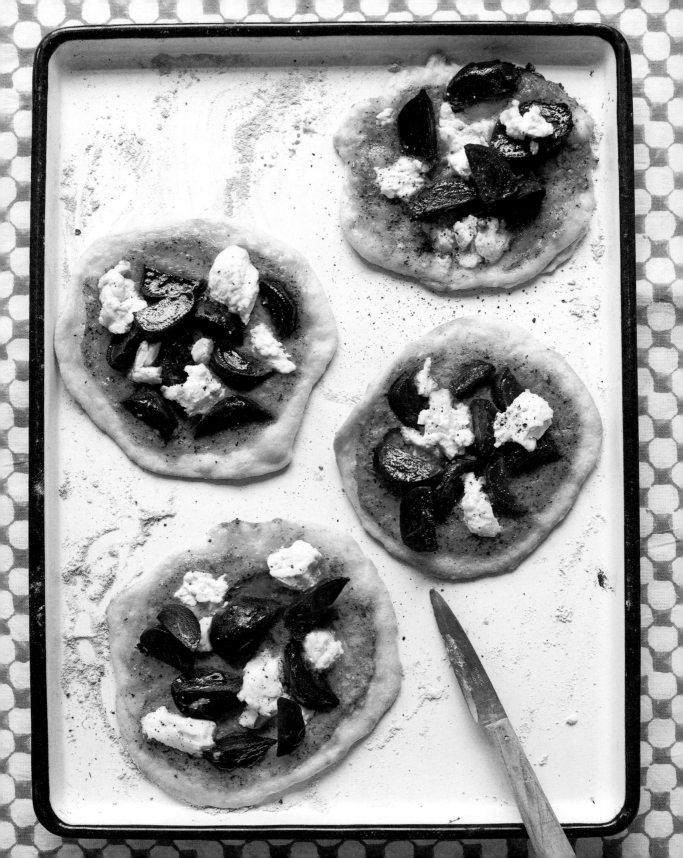

Nourishing butternut squash pie

Butternut squash is easy to digest, so this comparatively heavy dinner dish can be eaten early in the evening without placing a burden on the digestive system. Equally it could be enjoyed at lunch too, so feel free to double up the quantities and reheat a portion the next day for lunch, or take it out with you in a food flask. This is a good recipe to enjoy in the days following a three-day Seasonal Reset Ritual (see page 52).

Serves 2–3
Preparation time 5 minutes, plus soaking
Cooking time 1–1¼ hours

1 butternut squash, halved, deseeded and
  flesh scored
1 teaspoon ghee (see page 196) or olive oil
90g (3¼oz) mung beans, soaked overnight
1 litre (1¾ pints) boiling water
50g (1¾oz) brown rice
1 courgette, diced
1 leek, sliced into rings
2 teaspoons sweet paprika
small pinch of chopped fresh or dried thyme
pinch of dried or chopped fresh rosemary
handful of grated hard cheese
unrefined salt and black pepper

Preheat the oven to 200°C/180°C fan (400°F), Gas Mark 6.

Place the squash halves, with their cut sides facing up, on a baking tray. Cover with ½ teaspoon of the ghee or olive oil and bake for 40–60 minutes, until soft. Meanwhile, prepare the other components of the dish.

Drain the mung beans and put them into a saucepan with the measured boiling water. Simmer over a medium–low heat for 30 minutes.

Cook the rice in another pan according to the packet instructions.

Heat the remaining ghee in a medium saucepan over a medium–low heat. Add the courgette, leek, sweet paprika, thyme and rosemary and sauté gently for 6 minutes, until the vegetables are soft, adding a splash of water if necessary, to keep them moist.

Drain any excess liquid from both the cooked mung beans and the rice, then mix them into the cooked courgette and leek. Season with salt and pepper.

Scoop out the squash flesh from its skin into a bowl and mash it with a fork.

Arrange the bean mixture across the bottom of a 1 litre (1¾ pint) baking dish. Cover the surface with the mashed squash, then sprinkle over the grated cheese. Bake for 10–15 minutes, until the potato is slightly browned on top.

Tip
You can create many different versions of this recipe by substituting different beans for the mung beans and using seasonal vegetables for the filling.

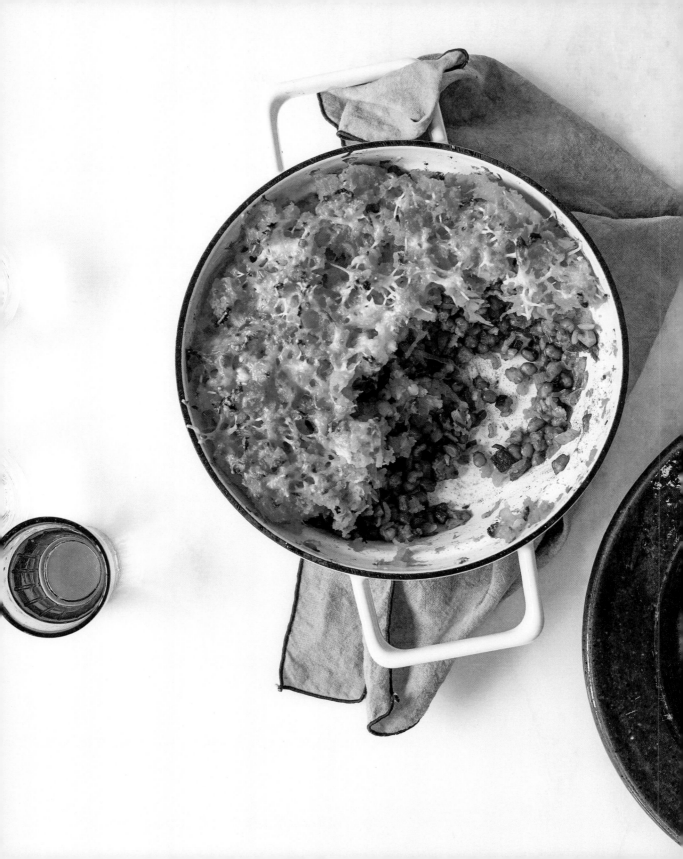

Sweetness and delight _____

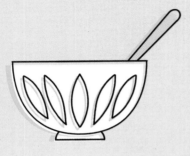

Desserts and sweet treats are a gift to both the physical body and our emotional senses, as sweetness offers comfort to a taxed nervous system. While, culturally, many of us consider sweet dishes something for after dinner, ideally your meals should be sufficient in quantity that there is no desire for a pudding, and sweet treats should be reserved for those times when you have been working hard and require something that will boost energy levels until the next meal.

This section contains treats that can be enjoyed mid-morning or mid-afternoon, along with desserts for special celebrations. The recipes either harness the natural sugars available in fruits or rely on the addition of a little unrefined sugar.

Fruits are very high in vitamins and minerals. If the fruit is eaten on its own or before a meal, these nutrients can be easily and quickly digested, as there is no digestive competition from other food sources. This means all of the fabulous nutrients can be quickly and easily assimilated, stored and utilized.

Puddings can be hard to digest, owing to their high fat and sugar content and the fact that they are normally blended with nutritious and sweet grains – you get sweet on sweet on sweet. When puddings are not digested properly, they promote the production of excess mucus in the body. If you suffer from lethargy after eating a large meal followed by a dessert, your body is telling you that the digestive system has been overburdened. But if desserts are eaten before a meal, when the digestive capacity is higher than at the end of the meal, the sugars and fats are often converted more efficiently. So, if you are serving treats alongside a meal, consider eating the sweet course first.

Tea time, time out

Mid to late afternoon can sometimes be an ideal time to take
some time out. Whether you can manage five or a full twenty
minutes to go 'offline', this break can be really helpful to
boost you for the rest of the afternoon/evening.

Take yourself to a quiet corner, either sit comfortably
or lie down flat on the floor in *Savasana* (corpse pose) and
close your eyes. Set an alarm if necessary and put on some
relaxing music or a 'yoga *nidra*' recording, and let yourself
be carried away. When you come round you should feel refreshed
and revived. Take a peek in the resources section at the
end of the book where you will find some of my favourite
recordings that have the right kind of *Naad* sound. Any gentle
instrumental music or other mantra music is good too — the
key is to find a sound that you like.

Gluten-free spiced cookies _____

Combining rice flour, which is sweet in nature, with astringent buckwheat flour creates a good balance in these deliciously spiced cookies. And the ghee combats the drying nature of the flours. Cinnamon is pungent, bitter, sweet and heating. It is also really good for oral health; you can simply chew on a tiny bit of cinnamon stick to benefit from its properties. Enjoy these cookies with a hot drink or try them topped with some nut butter. They are perfect for taking on journeys to provide an energy boost between meals.

Makes approximately 20 cookies
Preparation time 10 minutes
Cooking time 8–10 minutes

85g (3oz) ghee (see page 196), plus extra
   for greasing
50g (1¾oz) coconut sugar
½ teaspoon vanilla extract or seeds from
   ½ vanilla pod
½ teaspoon ground cinnamon
½ teaspoon ground ginger
½ teaspoon baking powder
pinch of unrefined salt
125g (4½oz) rice flour, plus extra for dusting
75g (2¾oz) buckwheat flour
2 tablespoons water

Preheat the oven to 200°C/180°C fan (400°F), Gas Mark 6. Grease and flour a baking sheet.

Put the ghee and sugar into a bowl and stir together with a wooden spoon for a minute to combine. Add the remaining ingredients and mix into a dough.

Dust your work top with flour. Using a rolling pin, roll out the dough to a thickness of 5mm (¼in). Use cookie cutters to cut out different shapes, as desired.

Transfer the dough shapes to the prepared baking sheet and bake for 8–10 minutes, until light golden brown. Transfer to a wire rack and leave to cool completely. Store in an airtight container.

Tip
Experiment to find your favourite spice combinations for these cookies. For instance, cardamom has similar properties to cinnamon but offers a very different flavour. Feel free to change the flours used too – try oat flour in place of the rice flour, for instance.

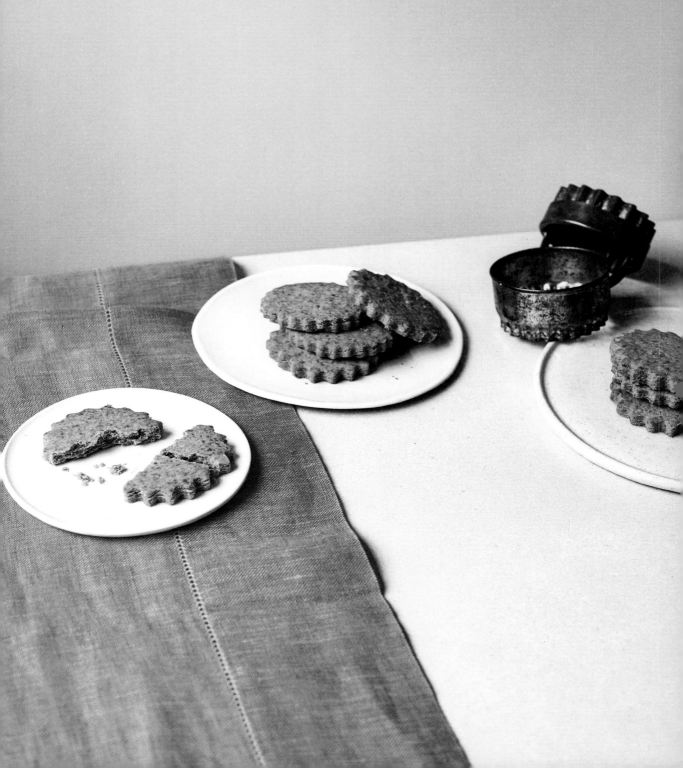

Anti-congestion spicy crackers _____

Consider these crispy crackers a medicinal treat – they are wonderful for when you have a runny nose or wet cough. The combination of ingredients is similar to those in a classic Ayurvedic remedy known as *sitopaladi*. Enjoy one in the morning before breakfast and one in the evening before dinner, to promote good digestion. Even if you are not suffering, you can have the crackers as preventative medicine, as they will bring balance to the body in damp and cold weather. For the benefits of amaranth, see opposite.

Makes 10 crackers
Preparation time 5 minutes
Cooking time 15 minutes

1½ tablespoons honey
⅛ teaspoon ground cinnamon
⅛ teaspoon ground cardamom
⅛ teaspoon ground white pepper or
  dried thyme
1 tablespoon sunflower seeds
15g (½oz) unrefined cane sugar
25g (1oz) amaranth

Before you begin, lay out a large sheet of baking paper on your work top. Combine the honey, spices and sunflower seeds in a bowl. Put the sugar into a separate bowl.

Heat a large saucepan over a medium–high heat for several minutes, until it is very hot. Put 1 tablespoon of the amaranth into the hot pan and immediately cover the pan with the lid. Shake the pan back and forth on the hob continuously – while you do, the amaranth will pop dramatically, just as popcorn does, but much more rapidly. As soon as the first portion has puffed, take the pan off the heat and tip the puffed amaranth into a bowl. Repeat the process, puffing small amounts of amaranth each time, until the total amount has been puffed.

Put the saucepan back on the hob over a low heat. Tip the sugar into the pan and heat it gently. As soon as it has melted, take the pan off the heat, wait for a few seconds, then add all the puffed amaranth and stir until the mixture is fully combined. Allow it to cool for a few moments, until it is cool enough to touch, then mix in the honey, spices and sunflower seeds.

Turn the mixture out onto one half of the prepared sheet of baking paper, then fold the other half of the paper over the mixture. Using a rolling pin, roll out the mixture between the two leaves of paper, to a thickness of 1cm (½in). Leave to firm up for 1 hour, then peel back the top layer of paper and cut the block into 2cm (¾in) squares. Store in an airtight container for up to 3 days on your countertop or in the larder.

Tip
These crackers pack a spicy punch, as they are designed to be taken when suffering from a cold. If you are not feeling unwell, but just enjoy aromatic flavours, omit the white pepper and enjoy the enticing flavours of cinnamon and cardamom.

Carob crackers

In these crackers, puffed amaranth is combined with chocolaty carob for a crispy treat. Amaranth, a heavenly ancient grain, is light, easy to digest and balancing for all constitutional types (see page 15). It is packed with minerals such as magnesium and manganese. Manganese is vital for bone development and enzyme activity.

Makes 10 crackers
Preparation time 5 minutes
Cooking time 15 minutes

25g (1oz) amaranth
2 tablespoons honey
½ tablespoon carob powder (or use cocoa powder)
1 tablespoon sunflower seeds

Before you begin, lay out a large sheet of baking paper on your work top.

Heat a large saucepan over a medium–high heat for several minutes until it is very hot. Put 1 tablespoon of the amaranth into the hot pan and immediately cover the pan with the lid. Shake the pan back and forth on the hob continuously – while you do, the amaranth will pop dramatically, just as popcorn does, but much more rapidly. As soon as the first portion has puffed, take the pan off the heat and tip the puffed amaranth into a bowl. Repeat the process, puffing small amounts of amaranth each time until the total amount has been puffed.

Take the saucepan off the heat and allow it to cool a little. When it is only just warm, add the honey and allow it to melt – this way, the honey remains uncooked. Mix in the carob powder thoroughly, then incorporate the sunflower seeds. Finally, add the puffed amaranth and stir until the mixture is combined.

Turn the mixture out onto one half of the prepared sheet of baking paper, then fold the other half over the mixture. Using a rolling pin, roll out the mixture between the two leaves of paper, to a thickness of 1cm (½in). Leave to firm up for 1 hour, then peel back the top layer of paper and cut the block into 2cm (¾in) squares. Store in an airtight container for up to 3 days on your countertop or in the larder, if they last that long!

Tips

• These crackers offer the perfect alternative to traditional chocolate crispy cake. They have a similar taste, but there is no high-to-low sugar swing that comes with it. If you cannot source amaranth, look for puffed rice and stir these into the melted honey mixture.

• If it is hot and your honey is very runny before cooking, put the crackers in the refrigerator to firm up after you have made them.

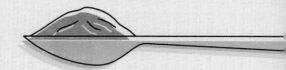

Mini-panforte

These mini-cakes are my Ayurvedic version of panforte, the classic chewy, self-preserving and highly portable Italian dessert traditionally made by monks in the 13th century. To negate any potential drying effect of the dried fruit, I add a little ghee. Traditionally fats were not added to panforte, but I think it works well. The crystallized ginger, in conjunction with the nutmeg, cardamom and cinnamon, produces a lovely warmth and helps you to process the natural sugars. The combination of the protein in the nuts and the sugars and dietary fibre from the figs, means these panforte are like fortified energy balls. To make a vegan and gluten-free version, replace the ghee with coconut oil and the flour with gluten-free flour.

Makes 10 mini cakes
Preparation time 10 minutes, plus cooling
Cooking time 25 minutes

75g (2¾oz) dried figs
75g (2¾oz) dried apricots
40g (1½oz) crystallized ginger, diced
40g (1½oz) walnuts, broken into pieces
40g (1½oz) whole hazelnuts
75g (2¾oz) white spelt flour
70g (2½oz) coconut sugar
15g (½oz) ghee (see page 196)
pinch of grated nutmeg
½ teaspoon ground cinnamon
seeds from 2 large green cardamom pods,
    ground to a powder

Preheat the oven to 170°C/150°C fan (340°F), Gas Mark 3½. Cut out 10 baking paper discs and use one to line 10 of the recesses of a 12-hole muffin tin.

Put the figs, apricots and crystallized ginger into a blender jug and blitz until smooth. If you do not have a blender, chop them finely with a knife.

Place the nuts on a baking tray and toast in the oven for 3–4 minutes, until they begin to brown. Combine the flour in a bowl with the nuts, once they are toasted.

Put the sugar, ghee and spices into a saucepan and cook over a medium heat, stirring with a wooden spoon, for roughly 5 minutes, until the sugar liquifies and the mixture looks like melted chocolate. This is a little tricky, as coconut sugar can become smoky quickly. As soon as the sugar has melted, quickly mix in the blended fruit, stirring vigorously with a wooden spoon. Take the pan off the heat and add the nuts and flour. Keep stirring until the mixture is well combined. Set aside to cool a little.

When the mixture is cool enough to handle, take a large spoonful of it, roll it into a ball between your palms and squash it into a disc roughly the size of a recess in your muffin tin. Place it in one of the lined recesses. Continue in this way until all the mixture is used up.

Bake for 15 minutes or until the mini-cakes take on a more golden colour. Leave to cool completely in the tins. The mixture will set and firm up on cooling. Store in an airtight container for up to 1 week.

Tips

- Ayurvedic mini-panforte make the ideal gift, especially for winter festivities. When you are ready to present them, take them out of their airtight container and wrap them up in beeswax cloth to keep them fresh, or use paper and ribbon.

- You can also use unrefined sugar in place of coconut sugar – it melts a little more easily than coconut sugar.

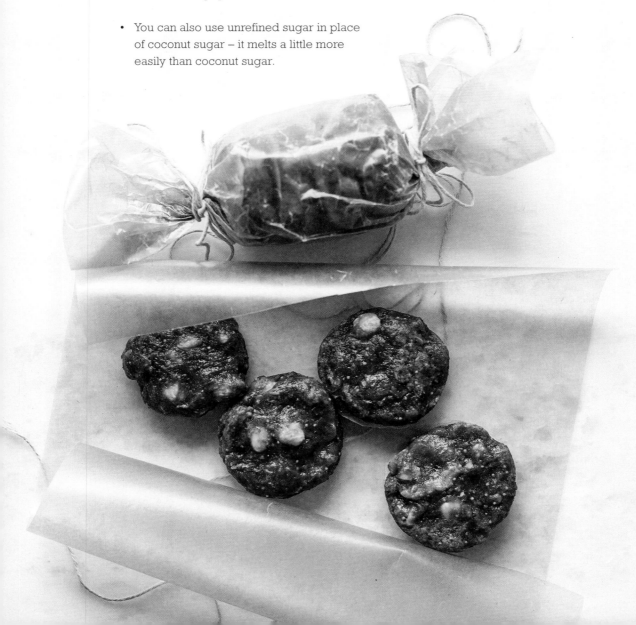

Soothing apple and blackberry crumblies _____

Each of these mini-crumblies is a mouthful of autumnal delight, but if you get organized, they can be a treat throughout the winter too. Blackberry picking is one of my favourite early autumn activities. Blackberries are jam packed with vitamins C and K, as well as antioxidants and micronutrients that will boost the immune system ahead of the winter. So, in the autumn, head to your nearest fruiting hedgerow and enjoy gathering the plump fruits while soaking up the last rays of summer sun, then wash and freeze your pickings.

Makes 12 mini-crumblies
Preparation time 12 minutes
Cooking time 25–30 minutes

2 dessert apples, peeled, cored and chopped
handful of sweet blackberries
100g (3½oz) spelt flour (or use oat flour or
    gluten-free flour), plus extra for dusting
40g (1½oz) wheatgerm (or replace with extra
    spelt flour)
40g (1½oz) ghee (see page 196), plus extra
    for greasing
¼ teaspoon ground ginger
agave nectar, maple syrup or honey, to serve
    (optional)

Preheat the oven to 200°C/180°C fan (400°F),
Gas Mark 6. Grease and flour each of the
recesses of a 12-hole muffin tin.

Put the apples, blackberries and a splash of
water into a small saucepan over a medium–
low heat. Cook down the fruit to a sauce-like
consistency – this should take 5–10 minutes.
Drain off any excess juice (you can drink this
– it is delicious).

Meanwhile, put the flour, wheatgerm, ghee
and ground ginger into a mixing bowl and
combine with your fingers until the mixture
has a crumb-like texture. Tip 1 tablespoon
of the crumble mixture into the base of each
recess in the prepared muffin tin. Press the
mixture firmly into the bottom of each recess
using the back of a spoon in order to create
a solid and level base.

Then, when the apple sauce is ready, spoon
1 tablespoon of it into each recess of the muffin
tin over the crumble base. Top with 1 more
tablespoon of the crumble mixture.

Bake for 20 minutes, until the tops are golden
brown. Remove from the oven and allow to
cool in the tin slightly, then carefully remove
each crumbly using a spatula. Serve warm
or cold. These are deliberately made to be
semi-sweet, so you can drizzle a tiny amount
of agave nectar, maple syrup or honey over
each crumbly before serving, if desired.

Tips
- Experiment with different seasonal fruit
  and flavouring combinations. Raspberry
  and pear work well together, as do
  apricots and cinnamon.

- To make a compote from leftover
  blackberries, follow the beginning of the
  recipe above, cooking the fruit to a sauce-
  like consistency, then stir in 2 tablespoons
  lemon juice and continue to cook for a
  further minute. Take the pan off the heat and
  leave the mixture to cool. When it is nearly
  cold, stir in honey to taste. Leave to cool
  completely, then transfer to a sterilized jar
  (see page 196 for sterilizing instructions),
  seal and refrigerate for up to 2 weeks.

Upfront energy balls

The warming fresh ginger in these energy balls perfectly balances the cooling coconut and date, making this a treat for all constitutional types (see page 15). This is an instantaneous energizing snack, for when you need a super-quick, supercharged boost. It is worth using Medjool dates in these energy balls – they are very gooey and yummy.

Makes approximately 15 balls
Preparation time 20 minutes

6 large Medjool dates or 200g (7oz) dried
   dates, pitted and finely chopped
25g (1oz) fresh root ginger, peeled and
   finely chopped
100g (3½oz) desiccated coconut

Line an airtight container with baking paper.

Put the ingredients into a mixing bowl and combine well to form a paste. You will need to use your hands to squeeze it all together, which can become a lovely mindful exercise.

Roll 1 tablespoon of the mixture into a ball between your palms. Place the ball in the prepared container and continue until you have used all the mixture up. Store in an airtight container in a refrigerator for up to 3 days. Bring to room temperature before eating.

Tips

• Omit the ginger if it is not to your taste or if you are prone to heating in your body. Alternatively, substitute crystallized ginger. It is less heating and enables you to store the balls for longer – they will keep for up to 1 week in an airtight container on your countertop or in the larder.

• Other nutritious ingredients can easily be incorporated into these energy balls. For instance, chopped sunflower seeds and pistachio nuts make excellent additions. For more local ingredients, substitute figs for dates and ground almonds for the coconut.

• Try rolling the balls in some cocoa powder mixed with salt for a real treat.

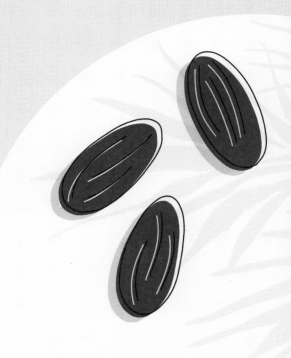

Pear crumble

Oats are full of fibre, help to lower bad cholesterol levels and provide long, slow, sustained energy. From an Ayurvedic viewpoint, oats are sweet and cooling, so combine well with warming cinnamon and allspice – and the combination tastes delicious too. This crumble is a bowl of sweet comfort, especially on a windy autumnal day.

Serves 4
Preparation time 10 minutes
Cooking time 25–30 minutes

4 pears, peeled, cored and chopped
115g (4oz) oat flour
115g (4oz) porridge oats
¼ teaspoon ground allspice
1 teaspoon ground cinnamon
75g (2¾oz) coconut sugar
75g (2¾oz) ghee (see page 196), at room
  temperature

Preheat the oven to 200°C/180°C fan (400°F), Gas Mark 6.

Arrange the chopped pears in the base of 1 litre (1¾ pint) baking dish.

Combine the remaining ingredients in a mixing bowl until the mixture reaches a crumb-like consistency. Sprinkle the topping over the pears. Bake for 25–30 minutes, until the crumble is golden brown. Serve warm or cold.

Tips
- If there happens to be any of this pudding left over, keep it refrigerated overnight, then enjoy it at room temperature the next morning for breakfast or as a snack.

- It's easy to make your own oat flour for this recipe. Simply place 115g (4oz) oats in a blender and whizz them up.

- You can substitute the Multi-grain Muesli on page 108 for the oats in this recipe. Use the same quantity.

- Experiment with different seasonal fruits for this dish. Try rhubarb in the spring (add some extra sugar to the rhubarb and some young angelica leaves, to mask the acidic taste); plums and greengages are delicious in summer; and apples and blackberries are ripe and juicy in the autumn and winter. Firmer fruits such as apples and rhubarb will need precooking on the stove first.

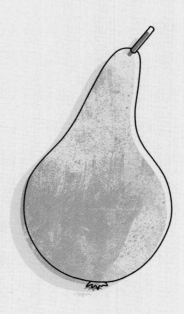

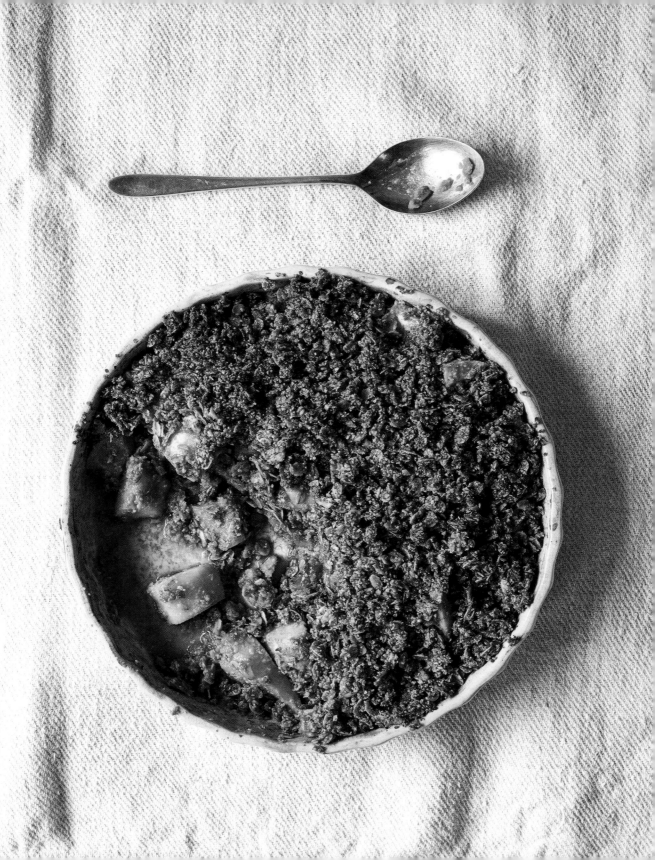

Vegan pumpkin pie

This dish is almost a meal in itself. It is not overly sweet and makes a great dessert before a meal (see page 162). This combination of pumpkin and spices is ideal in autumn, as it helps to cleanse the heat of the summer out of the body. Pumpkin is rich in vitamin A, which is essential for good eyesight and efficient immunity.

Serves 6–8
Preparation time 10 minutes, plus cooling
Cooking time 1 hour 20 minutes

For the pastry
150g (5½oz) spelt flour, plus extra for dusting
4 tablespoons mild olive oil, plus extra
   for greasing
50ml (2fl oz) water
⅛ teaspoon unrefined salt

For the filling
375g (13oz) pumpkin, peeled, deseeded
   and diced
4 tablespoons water
3 tablespoons cornflour
1 tablespoon olive oil
100ml (3½fl oz) almond milk
30g (1oz) coconut sugar
½ teaspoon ground ginger
1 teaspoon ground cinnamon
¼ teaspoon grated nutmeg
2 ground cloves

Preheat the oven to 200°C/180°C fan (400°F), Gas Mark 6. Grease a 24cm (9½in) tart tin.

Put the pumpkin in a saucepan with the measured water and cook over a low heat until soft – this can take between 10 and 20 minutes.

Meanwhile, make the pastry. Sift the flour into a bowl, then add the olive oil, measured water and salt and bring the mixture together with your hands to form a dough.

Dust your work top with flour. Using a rolling pin, roll out the dough into a circle with a diameter of roughly 24cm (9½in). Carefully transfer the dough to the prepared tart tin. If it cracks or tears, use your hands to mould and shape it into the tin, compressing it to close any gaps and give it a smooth, seamless finish. Bake in the oven for 5 minutes while you prepare the filling.

Place the cooked pumpkin and the remaining filling ingredients into a blender jug and blitz until smooth.

Remove the tart tin from the oven, pour in the filling, then bake for 1 hour, until it is golden on the top. Carefully touch the top of the pie – if it feels firm, it is ready. Allow to cool before serving.

Tips
- This pie can be made the day before serving, if you are short of time. Store in the refrigerator overnight and remove it an hour before serving, to allow it to come up to room temperature.

- Butternut squash can be substituted for pumpkin (as can different flours for spelt). It requires a longer initial cooking time than the pumpkin, in plenty of water.

Carrot and beetroot celebration cake _____

This cake is grounding and nourishing, and is not too heavy on the digestive system, as it uses sunflower oil, which is a lighter fat than butter. The honey helps to balance any mucus-promoting traits of the labneh (see page 201) or cream cheese filling. The flavour of labneh is sourer than that of the cream cheese, so choose which to use according to your taste.

Serves 8
Preparation time 10 minutes, plus cooling
Cooking time 30–45 minutes

175ml (6fl oz) sunflower oil, plus extra
  for greasing
150g (5½oz) coconut sugar
4 eggs
2 carrots, peeled and grated
1 beetroot, peeled and grated
1 teaspoon vanilla bean paste
2 teaspoons ground cinnamon
75g (2¾oz) walnuts, lightly crushed
200g (7oz) self-raising gluten-free flour,
  plus extra for dusting
1 teaspoon baking powder

For the filling
200g (7oz) mascarpone cheese or labneh
  (see page 201)
2 tablespoons honey
finely grated zest of 1 unwaxed orange
whole walnuts, to decorate

Preheat the oven to 200°C/180°C fan (400°F), Gas Mark 6. Grease and flour 2 × 18cm (7in) cake tins.

Put the oil, sugar and eggs into a mixing bowl and whisk together for a few minutes, until frothy. Fold in the carrot, beetroot, vanilla paste, cinnamon and walnuts. Finally, fold in the flour and baking powder to form a light batter.

Divide the mixture between the prepared cake tins, then bake for 30–45 minutes, until a skewer inserted into the centre of each cake comes out clean. Turn the cake layers out onto wire racks and leave to cool.

When the cake layers are cool, make the topping. Put the ingredients into a mixing bowl and whisk to combine them thoroughly.

Place a cake layer on a serving plate and spread half of the filling across the surface. Carefully place the next cake layer on top, then spread the remaining filling mixture over. Decorate with whole walnuts to serve.

Tips
• To make your own labneh for the topping, follow the recipe on page 201, omitting the cumin.

• Feel free to experiment with other vegetables for this cake. For instance, similar quantities of sweet potato or butternut squash can be used in place of the carrot and beetroot. Add some chopped stem ginger and ¼ teaspoon of ground ginger if you are feeling like you could do with some additional warmth.

Nourishing almond and cardamom polenta cake _____

Desserts notoriously encourage sluggishness within the digestive system and can fuel certain imbalances within the body. To counter this, I have made this cake low in sugar and use polenta and gluten-free flour, which are lighter in nature than wheat flour. The turmeric and cardamom in the spiced cream help reduce the cream's mucus-enhancing trait. The end result is more like a pudding than a sponge cake, with a crumbly, nutty texture that is delightful with the warm spiced cream.

Serves 8–10
Preparation time 15 minutes, plus cooling
Cooking time 40 minutes

100g (3½oz) ghee (see page 196) or
   sunflower oil
100g (3½oz) coconut sugar or unrefined
   cane sugar
4 eggs
125g (4½oz) gluten-free flour
75g (2¾oz) ground almonds
140g (5oz) polenta
2 teaspoons baking powder
seeds from 4 cardamom pods, ground using
   a pestle and mortar
250ml (9fl oz) almond milk (see page 190)
seeds from 1 vanilla pod or ½ teaspoon
   vanilla essence

For the spiced cream
125ml (4fl oz) double cream
¼ teaspoon turmeric
3 cardamom pods, gently crushed and opened

Preheat the oven to 200°C/180°C fan (400°F), Gas Mark 6. Line a 23cm (9in) round cake tin with baking paper.

Put the ghee and sugar into a bowl and stir together with a wooden spoon for a minute to combine. Then mix in the eggs and the dry ingredients. Thin the mixture using the almond milk to create a batter with a dropping consistency, then stir in the vanilla.

Pour the batter into the prepared cake tin and bake for 40 minutes, until a skewer inserted into the centre of the cake comes out clean. Toward the end of the cooking time, watch the cake carefully and, at approximately 30 minutes, if the top begins to look too dark, cover the tin with some kitchen foil to prevent burning. When the cake is baked, remove it from the oven, turn it out onto a wire rack and leave to cool.

Once the cake has cooled, make the fragrant spiced cream sauce. Pour the cream into a saucepan set over a low heat, stir in the spices and bring the mixture to a boil slowly, stirring occasionally. As soon as the cream begins to boil gently, take the pan off the heat and leave to cool a little. This will help the spices infuse the cream and give it a golden colour.

When ready to serve, cut the cake into slices and serve each slice with the warm cream poured over.

Tips

- This recipe is versatile, so experiment with your favourite ingredients. Try using ground hazelnuts or pistachios instead of almonds. Both are sweet, heating and energizing. Rose water can be used instead of vanilla – omit the cardamom pods and decorate the top with edible rose petals after cooling.

- You could also make a rose cream, mixing a little rosewater into a non-dairy cream, omitting the turmeric and cardamom. Rose is cooling, calming and emotionally soothing.

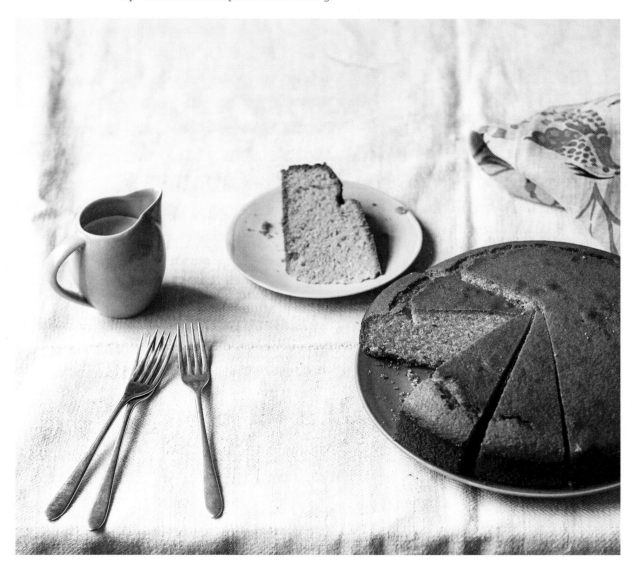

Drinks

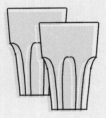

Drinks refresh and hydrate you and can be used to promote health, whether that be to calm you before bed, kick-start your digestive system, boost iron levels or help to alkalize an over-acidic stomach. Your taste preference is always of number-one importance, so feel free to switch up the ingredients and brewing times to make yourself the perfect beverage.

Ayurveda generally recommends sipping room temperature and/or warm drinks throughout the day, according to your thirst. Some of the infusions in this section can be enjoyed every day, such as the Nettle Leaf and Green Tea on page 183. Others are for more occasional use, when you feel like enjoying a particular taste or are looking for a specific health-promoting quality.

The total amount of liquid each person should consume throughout the day varies in relation to the ambient temperature and level of fluid loss through sweating (and, therefore, the level of activity). On average though, most adults should be drinking between six and eight glasses of water throughout the day, which may increase with temperature and activity rate. See the example opposite as a rough guide of an average day's fluid intake.

If you struggle to keep track of how much you drink, use the same 500ml (18fl oz) flask all day. Keeping it by your side gives you a visual prompt to encourage you to drink, and you can use it to help you keep track of how much you are drinking each day.

Daily fluid consumption — example

Use this example of daily fluid intake as a rough guide
for your own fluid consumption:

* 1 cup of hot water with a slice of lemon on waking

* 1 juice in the morning before breakfast or mid-morning,
  if you have been active and need a boost to carry you
  through until lunchtime

* 2 cups of Nettle Leaf and Green Tea (see page 183)
  throughout the morning and afternoon

* 2—4 cups of plain hot water or room-temperature water,
  with or without a slice of lemon or fresh mint

* 1 cup of Digestion-soothing Infusion (see page 180)
  15—20 minutes after a meal

* 1 milky drink in the evening before bed (unless you have a
  weak bladder, in which case have this earlier in the evening).

Digestion-soothing infusion _____

This tea is often known in the world of Ayurveda as CCF tea, which makes it easy to remember the ingredients – cumin, coriander and fennel seeds. If your digestive system is sluggish, and you often feel gassy after eating, take this refreshing drink after lunch or dinner. It prevents gas production and helps to release any trapped gas caused by poor digestive capacity or inappropriate diet. It also helps the body shift accumulated *ama* (metabolic waste).

Serves 2
Preparation time 3 minutes

¼ teaspoon fennel seeds
¼ teaspoon cumin seeds
¼ teaspoon coriander seeds
200ml ($^1/_3$ pint) water at 80°C (175°F)

Put the seeds into a small teapot and pour over the measured boiling water. Infuse for 3 minutes, then strain into a mug and serve.

Tips

- Chamomile flowers are a lovely addition to this mixture. Like the seeds used, chamomile is a cooling carminative. Not everyone likes the taste of chamomile, but adding it to this blend can mask its taste slightly. Try adding 1–3 small flower heads, depending on your taste preference. Chamomile is considered to be a *sattvic* herb (see page 14), bringing harmony to the body and mind. This tea is much less heating and stimulating than Green Chai (see page 182).

- It is easy to grow chamomile flowers in a pot. Fennel and coriander also make good pot plants, which, when ignored, easily produce seeds.

- The blend above, with or without the addition of chamomile, also supports a healthy monthly cycle.

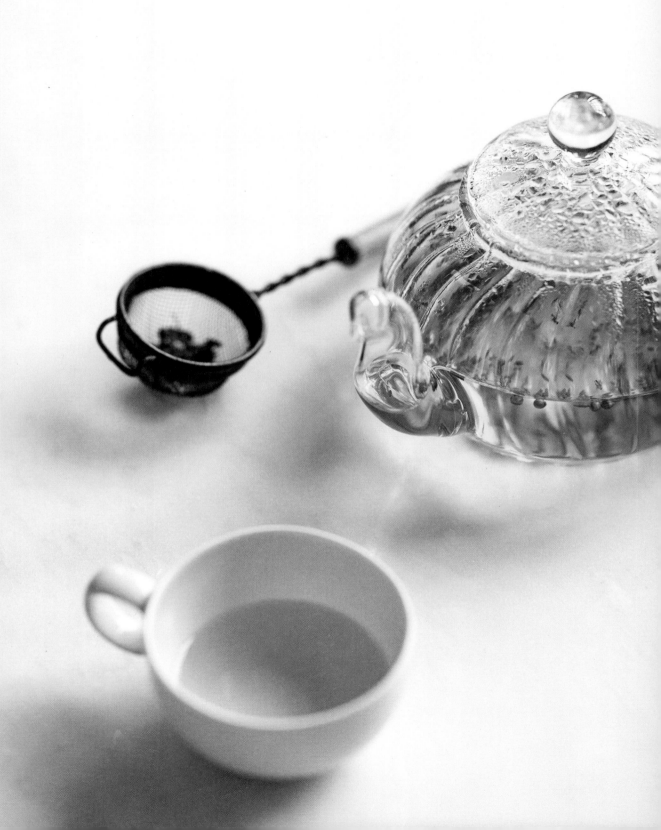

Green chai

If you are someone who generally feels cold, with cold hands and feet, and who has slow or erratic digestion, this is the drink for you, because the combination of spices is not overly heating, just warming, and green tea promotes good blood circulation. Green tea is also good for the brain, supporting cognition, as well as for the digestive system generally. It contains a third of the caffeine found in black tea, so is a great choice if you are looking to reduce your caffeine intake. The caffeine in coffee interrupts the signals in melatonin, the hormone that makes us sleepy and helps to regulate our circadian rhythms. Green tea contains a different type of caffeine that works by stimulating the limbic system instead, giving us an overall feeling of wakefulness without interrupting our sleep-wake cycle. Drink this tea 15 minutes after a meal if you have been eating something heavy, or anytime during the morning or early afternoon in the winter or if you are generally feeling cold. If you require a sweetener, add stevia.

Serves 2
Preparation time 15 minutes
Cooking time 7 minutes

1 teaspoon chopped fresh root ginger
3 cardamom pods
1 thin cinnamon stick
3 cloves
1 black peppercorn
700ml (1¼ pints) water
1 teaspoon green tea leaves

Place all the ingredients, except the green tea leaves, in a small saucepan, bring to a boil, then simmer over a medium–high heat for 7 minutes, until the water has begun to turn a light copper colour and the room is full of the aroma of the spices.

Meanwhile, put the green tea leaves into a small teapot.

Take the pan off the heat and allow to cool for 6–7 minutes, until the temperature has reduced to 70–80°C (160–175°F). Pour it into the teapot containing the tea leaves and leave the tea to infuse for 3–4 minutes, then pour into a mug and serve.

Tips

- Do feel free to adjust the spices/tea leaves/cooking time to your preference. I recommend substituting white tea for the green tea.

- For a quick warming drink, use just one of the spices. For example, put into a tea strainer just a few tiny pieces of cinnamon with ½ teaspoon chopped fresh root ginger, and ½ teaspoon green tea leaves and place the strainer in a mug. Pour over 200ml (¹/₃ pint) water at 70°C (160°F) and leave to infuse for 4 minutes before drinking.

- Add ½ chopped lemon grass stalk to this recipe to aid digestion further.

Nettle leaf and green tea

This combination is an immune-boosting power cup. As well as being a tonic for the blood when drunk daily, it also supports the urinary system and has a mild diuretic action. Green tea contains a lot of health-promoting amino acids. Theanine in particular boosts cognitive brain function. Nettles are full of nutrients, especially vitamins A and C, iron, potassium and calcium. The temperature used when processing nettle leaves is important. The optimum amount of vitamin C is extracted when the leaves are steeped at 50–60°C (122–140°F) for 10 minutes.

Makes 1 dose
Preparation time 10 minutes

2 teaspoons dried or fresh organic nettle leaves
1 teaspoon loose-leaf high-quality green tea
500ml (18fl oz) water at 50–60°C (122–140°F)

Place the leaves in a tea strainer and cover with the measured hot water. Leave to infuse for up to 10 minutes, then serve immediately.

Tips
• One of the signs that spring has arrived is the new growth of nettles, which continue to grow through the summer and into the late autumn. In the spring you can don rubber gloves and collect nettles for washing and drying or dehydrating, ready for storage and use throughout the year. Your growing vegetables and herbs love nettle extract too – pull up unwanted nettles, leave them to fester in some water for a couple of weeks, then pour that water over the growing soil and look forward to a bumper crop!

• A 100g (3½oz) portion of steamed young nettle leaves can provide 90–100 per cent of your recommended daily intake of vitamin A, which is essential for good eye health and nerve conduction. They can be used like any other greens – try adding them to soups and stews.

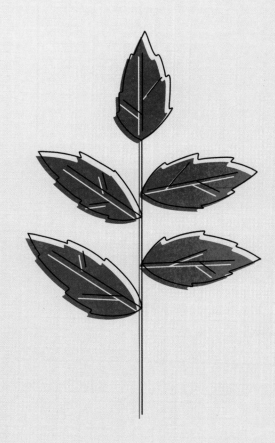

Cooling cucumber and celery juice ————————————

This cooling, soothing juice is fabulous for an over-heated digestive system, and the lettuce it contains helps to relax the nervous system. Drink it at the height of the summer to quench your thirst. The summer is a great time of year to enjoy juices. According to Ayurveda, unless a person is blessed with a naturally strong digestive system, juices are considered to be too cooling for the digestive system when it is very cold outside, unless they are made naturally heating with the use of ginger and other warming additives. In the summer, our calorific needs are less and juices are a great way to introduce quick nourishment. And, as the cellulose structures in the vegetables are broken down, so the vitamins and minerals can be quickly absorbed.

Serves 1
Preparation time 5 minutes

$^1/_3$ cucumber or 20 black or red grapes
2 celery sticks
4 lettuce leaves

Scrub the vegetables and cut them down to size if necessary, to fit through the feeder chute of your juicer. Then push the ingredients through the juicer one by one. Enjoy immediately.

Tip
If you are feeling the cold but like the idea of something refreshing, opt for the black or red grapes instead of cucumber and add ½ teaspoon chopped fresh ginger. Black grapes can help when you feel as though you have a hot head or unquenchable thirst (in which case omit the ginger).

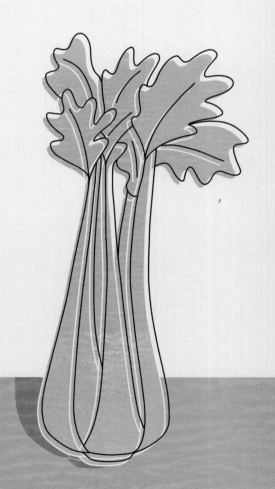

Iron-promoting juice _____

Feeling exhausted can make you feel blue. This juice is particularly supportive if your energy levels are low, especially due to a reduced iron count. Its invitingly sweet flavour makes this drink a nourishing treat. Beetroot is rich in folate and iron, but iron from plant sources needs vitamin C present in order for the body to be able to absorb it. Beetroot contains some vitamin C but, in this drink, more is added with the inclusion of apples and carrots. From an Ayurvedic perspective, the apples and beetroot are cooling, while the carrot and ginger are warming, creating a nice blend.

Serves 1
Preparation time 5 minutes

1 beetroot
1 carrot
2 dessert apples
1cm (½in) piece of fresh root ginger

Scrub the vegetables and apples well and cut them down if necessary, to fit through the feeder chute of your juicer. Then push the ingredients through the juicer one by one. Enjoy immediately.

Tip
The consumption of juices during the colder months is not recommended in Ayurveda. In the winter, in order to feel warm within ourselves, it is helpful to consume foods that are warming in temperature and flavour, so a soup instead of a juice. However, ginger is included in this drink, so if you do desire a juice in the winter, this is a good one to try, as it has a warm feeling.

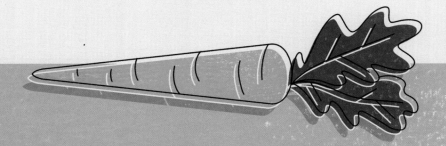

Night-time rose water and nutmeg milk _____

Rose water is soothing and calming, especially at times when you feel as though you could do with extra emotional support. Nutmeg has sedative properties and is slightly heating, but its warming quality is counterbalanced by the rose. Drinking a milky drink such as this one half an hour before bedtime can invoke a lovely feeling of comfort, helping to induce a good night's sleep.

Serves 1
Preparation time 5 minutes
Cooking time 2 minutes

200ml (¹/₃ pint) almond milk (see page 190)
   or dairy milk
2–3 drops of rose water or 1 teaspoon dried
   rose petals
tiny pinch of ground or grated nutmeg

Put the milk into a small saucepan and heat gently over a low heat until you see steam rising from it, then take the pan off the heat and allow to cool a little.

Stir in the rose water and nutmeg and leave to infuse for 5 minutes. Pour the infused milk (through a sieve if you are using petals) into a mug. Sit back and slowly sip the milk, allowing it to calm and settle you.

Tips

- Oat milk works well too, as a nut-free milk, and has lovely calming properties.

- Avoid any temptation to sweeten this drink if you are having it before bed. Sugar creates quick-release energy, which is likely to affect you just as you are about to close your eyes. Almond and dairy milk both contain natural sugars that do not create an energy spike, so try to become accustomed to their naturally sweet tastes.

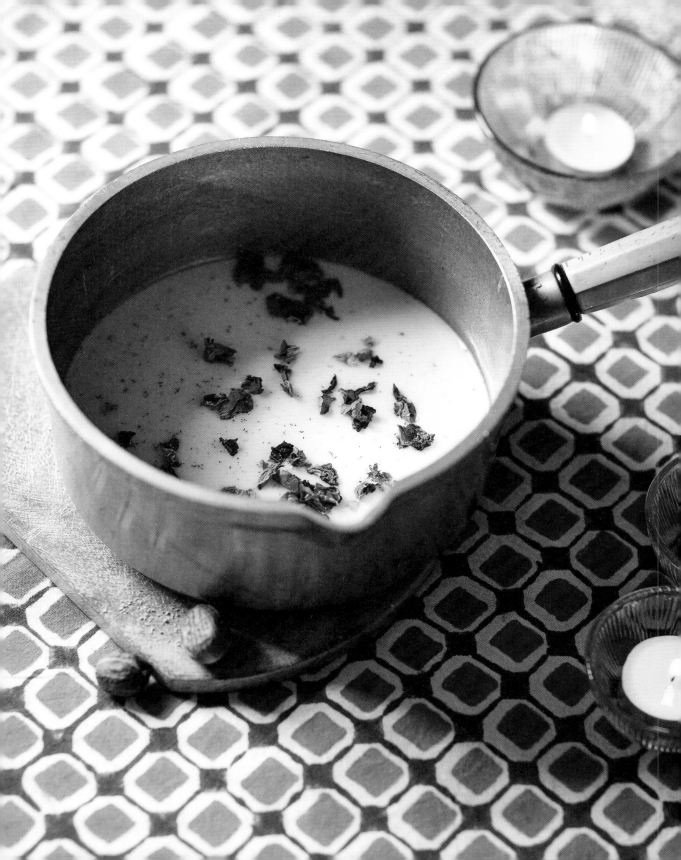

Alkalizing green juice _____

Acid can cause much discomfort. If you want to alkalize your digestive system gently, try this juice. The celery, greens and fennel help to clear out stagnation in the skin and urinary system. This cleansing juice has a delicate and clear flavour, perfect for those days when you are feeling hot and bothered.

Serves 1
Preparation time 5 minutes

1 carrot
2 celery sticks
¼ fennel bulb
1 apple
handful of leafy greens, such as beetroot
    tops or seasonal salad greens

Scrub the vegetables and apples well and cut them down if necessary, to fit through the feeder chute of your juicer. Then push the ingredients through the juicer one by one. Enjoy immediately.

Tips

- If you are feeling really hot and bothered in the summer, especially in the urinary system (with symptoms similar to those of cystitis), add a handful of fresh coriander leaves to the ingredients for this juice.

- To boost the alkalizing nature of the juice, stir 1 teaspoon spirulina or chlorella into the juice before drinking. These are both great blood tonics and are very alkalizing.

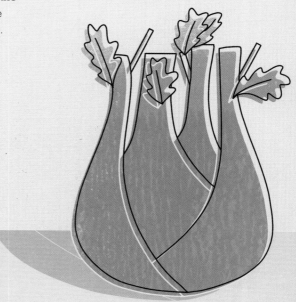

Good bacteria-boosting yogurt smoothie _____

When your digestive system needs a kick-start to relieve bloating, gas or IBS-type symptoms, try this savoury smoothie before lunch or dinner. The friendly bacteria in the yogurt and the gas-relieving properties of the cumin help prime the various segments of the digestive system for the coming meal. Make sure you use yogurt that contains live cultures, and look out for Greek yoghurt, which contains more protein than natural yogurt. The influence of the cumin, and the fact that you are taking the drink before the meal, means that the protein from the yogurt will be well absorbed by the body.

Serves 1
Preparation time 1 minute

4 tablespoons full-fat organic Greek yogurt
 or keffir yogurt
¼ teaspoon cumin seeds, ground with a
 pestle and mortar
150ml (¼ pint) warm water

Stir the ingredients together in a glass and serve immediately.

Tips

• If you have a low appetite, to avoid ruining it, take no more than half the quantity of this drink before your meal until your appetite has increased.

• Use yogurt to make a delicious dip that you can have as an appetizer with some vegetable crudités. Mix 100g (3½oz) yogurt with 1 teaspoon cumin seeds, lightly crushed.

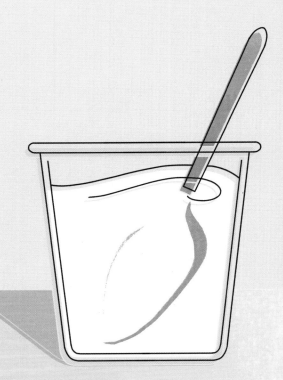

Homemade nut milk

Almonds are highly nourishing for the reproductive system and their high vitamin E content helps to give lustre to the skin and hair. Drinking this smooth almond milk allows quick absorption of the components with these properties. You could also make a hazelnut milk, using the same quantity of hazelnuts.

Serves 1
Preparation time 5 minutes, plus soaking

50g (1¾oz) almonds, soaked overnight
200ml (⅓ pint) water

Drain the soaked nuts, then remove the skins with your fingers – they should just slip off.

Place the skinned almonds in a blender jug with the measured water and blitz until smooth.

Line a sieve with muslin (cheesecloth), if you have any, and set this over a bowl. Tip the contents of the blender jug into the lined sieve and allow the liquid to drain through. (Reserve the almond pulp left behind for adding to porridge.) Drink immediately.

If you would like to use the almond milk for cooking, transfer it to a sterile glass bottle (see page 196 for sterilizing instructions) and refrigerate for up to 2 days.

Tip
If you miss the opportunity to soak the nuts and would like to make this milk in a hurry, put the almonds into a heatproof bowl and pour over very hot water to cover completely. Leave the nuts to soak for 30 minutes until plumped up. After this time, you should be able to rub away the skins with your fingers.

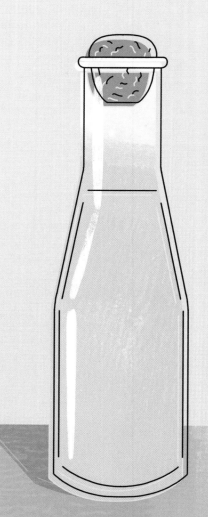

Ojas-boosting almond and saffron shake _____

Ojas is defined in Ayurveda as being what provides us with our immunity, reproductive excellence and longevity. This shake is highly nutritious and fortifying for body and mind. Many of the ingredients are considered to increase libido. Sesame seeds are a fantastic source of calcium and should be included regularly in the diet, especially for those who are dairy free. Saffron has wonderful mood-enhancing and anxiety-quelling[5] qualities. If you have been exerting yourself physically, this shake serves as a nice pick-me-up.

Serves 1
Preparation time 2 minutes
Cooking time 7 minutes

250ml (9fl oz) almond milk (see page 190)
    or dairy milk
1 teaspoon sesame seeds
tiny pinch ground ginger
3 saffron strands
4 small or 2 large pitted dates, finely chopped

Place all the ingredients in a saucepan, bring to simmering point, then simmer for 5 minutes.

Allow to cool a little, then drink warm or at room temperature. If you have a blender and prefer your drink to have a smooth consistency, once the mixture has cooled a little, transfer it to a blender jug and blitz before serving.

Tips

• As a nourishing tonic or *rasayana* (a rejuvenating preparation), take this drink once per day for a week.

• This milk can occasionally be fortified by adding some shatavari, a herb with sweet, bitter and cooling properties, or ashwagandha powder, which has sweet, astringent, bitter and heating properties. Add ½ teaspoon of your chosen herb into the saucepan. If you have been experiencing much stress lately and your nervous system has been particularly taxed, or if you need to improve your sleep quality, consider the benefits of ashwagandha. Shatavari (only to be used occasionally) is a good choice particularly for women, as it supports the reproductive system, including during menopause. It is also useful to men with a low sperm count. These variations of the shake are a nod to the Ayurvedic remedy known as Shatavari Kalpana, which works wonders for painful, irregular or absent periods. Either herb is suitable for both men and women, and they can be combined in one drink, in which case, use ¼ teaspoon of each.

Staples and condiments _____

This section contains recipes for staple ingredients (notably Ghee, see page 196) that are used in other recipes in this book. Some of these ingredients can be sourced readily in shops, but making them can be fun, satisfying and potentially more nutritious, owing to the control you can exert over the quality and freshness of the ingredients used to make the products. If you can afford the time to make these staples, it will be well spent.

This section also includes recipes for condiments to accompany a meal. These you would be hard pressed to buy, as they are not commonly available, but a dollop of one of these delicacies, such as Sprouted Chickpea Hummus (see page 200), adds another dimension on your plate. The beauty with the Spiced Pumpkin Jam (see page 197) and Ginger, Red Cabbage and Beetroot Sauerkraut (see page 194) is that they keep for a long time, so you can make them at the end of a growing season with a glut of produce and enjoy them throughout the next season.

Some of these recipes involve some kitchen alchemy, in the sense that they take an ingredient in one form and change it into a completely new form, with different properties and constituents. For example, ghee is made from heated butter. Nothing is added to it, yet the ghee's properties are changed through the cooking process: butter mildly increases acidity, whereas ghee acts as an antacid; butter builds *kapha* (see page 14) with its lactose solids, so is better suited to children and the elderly, whereas ghee helps to produce good cholesterol, is more or less lactose free, and does not increase *kapha*, so is better for adults. Also, butter has a lower smoke point that ghee. I find this alchemical process quite mesmerizing when I stop to think about it. These new properties are very health-promoting. It is certainly worth putting the time and energy into bringing them to life.

Easy peasy pickles

Most vegetables can be turned into pickle with little effort.

I like to use apple cider vinegar with 5 per cent acidity; with its sour taste it stimulates *agni* digestive fire. You can combine all sorts of vegetables and spices to create a full six-taste profile — just use your intuition and imagination to guide you as to flavour combinations. Alternately, choose your ingredients from the table below. If you suffer from inflammation conditions, however, keep pickle consumption low.

Chop your vegetables in any style you like and sprinkle them lightly with salt, then leave to rest in a bowl for a few hours — this helps preserve their texture. In a saucepan, bring to a simmer enough vinegar for your chosen jar, along with sweetener and spices. Cook the mixture for 2–3 minutes to release the flavours in the spices, then allow to cool.

Lift the vegetables out of the bowl and pack them into a sterilized jar (see page 196 for sterilizing instructions). Discard any leftover juices in the bowl. Pour over the spiced vinegar to cover the vegetables well. Secure the lid, label the jar and refrigerate once opened.

Pickle ingredients

Raw vegetables, chopped (enough to fill a jar)

cauliflower, cabbage

radishes

cucumber, courgette

carrots, thinly sliced beetroot

onion, shallots, spring onions

peppers

Sweetener (0–2 tablespoons)

maple syrup

unrefined cane sugar

honey (added after the vinegar has been heated)

Spices (½ teaspoon – 2 tablespoons)

fennel, coriander, cumin, celery, fenugreek and mustard seeds

peppercorns, juniper berries

bay leaves

fresh or dried green herbs

peeled garlic cloves

finely sliced fresh ginger, turmeric

Ginger, red cabbage and beetroot sauerkraut

A small amount of this tangy sauerkraut can be served alongside many dishes. Its sourness helps to boost gastric secretions and get the digestive system revving, and the many probiotic cultures that develop in it, especially those from the lactobacillus family[6], boost its function. These cultures may help to top up what may be dwindling populations for you, thus boosting the capacity of your digestive system. It is thought that 90 per cent of serotonin, the 'happy hormone', is made in our guts, so it is important that gut health is kept on top form. Your immunity also benefits from this sauerkraut. It is full of antioxidants that develop during fermentation, ready to boost your immune system throughout the winter. The longer you leave it to ferment, the stronger (sourer) it will be, and the more it will increase *pitta* (see page 14). I have recommended 5–7 days as an optimal time for most people.

Makes 400g (14oz)
Preparation time 15 minutes
Ferment time 1 week

350g (12oz) red cabbage, shredded (clean, trim and retain some outer leaves)
150g (5½oz) beetroot, grated
25g (1oz) fresh root ginger, peeled and grated
10g (¼oz) ground unrefined salt
½ teaspoon black mustard seeds

Place all the ingredients in a large bowl. Using both your hands, lift and squeeze the cabbage and beetroot repeatedly, coating the grated veg in the flavourings. After a few minutes, lots of liquid will be released.

Keep going until you feel as though the maximum liquid has been released from the vegetables.

Spoon some of the mixture into a sterile glass container (I use empty jam jars – see page 196 for sterilizing instructions), then use the end of a rolling pin or something similar to press the veg down inside the container, compacting it into the bottom of the jar. Continue adding 1 spoonful of the cabbage mixture at a time, pressing it down between each addition, until the cabbage reaches three-quarters of the way up the jar. Add liquid from the bowl into the jar to cover the veg and stop 2cm (¾in) below the top of the jar. Trim one of the reserved outer cabbage leaves to a circle slightly larger than the circumference of the jar you are using. Push this into the top of the liquid to form a lid. (This cabbage-leaf plug will prevent mould formation on the cabbage beneath, and can be discarded at a later date when you begin to use the product.) Screw on the lid and leave to ferment on the countertop away from sunlight.

Every day, unscrew the lid of the jar to release built-up gasses. Continue this process for 5–7 days. You can now taste the sauerkraut – when it gets to the point at which you like the level of its sourness, store it in the refrigerator, where it will keep for up to six months.

Tip
This is a great posture-breath-movement workout recipe (see page 38). You can really connect with the cabbage as you squeeze it, and feel as though you have got deeply involved in the process and put your energy and spirit into it.

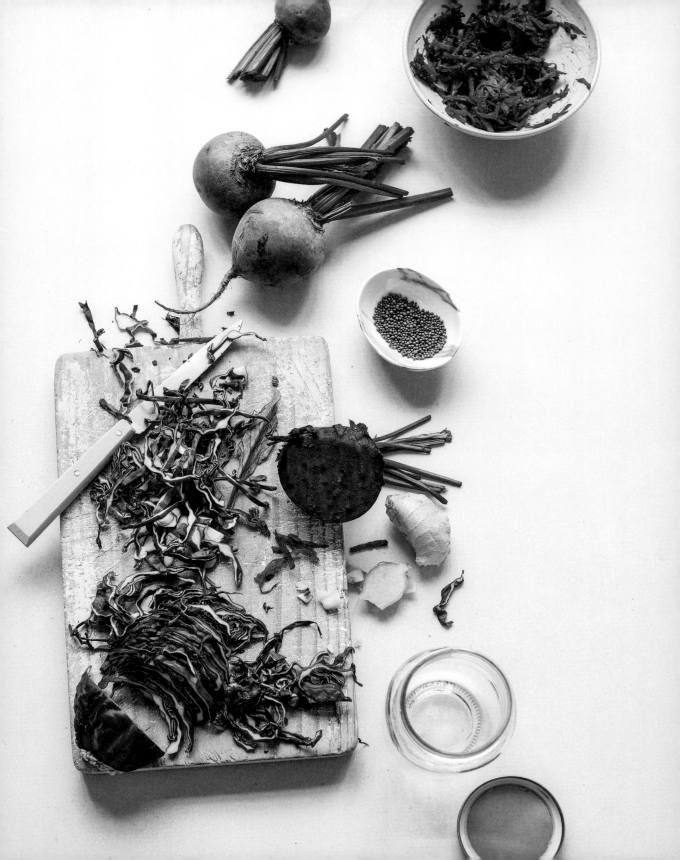

Ghee (clarified butter) _____

Ghee is prized in India as a superior cooking fat. It imparts a sweet flavour to food. According to Ayurveda, ghee helps to give elasticity to the skin and suppleness to the hair. When used in moderation, it contributes towards maintaining good cholesterol in the body. Ghee is simple to make, stores well and has many uses.

Makes 200g (7oz)
Preparation time 3 minutes
Cooking time 10–15 minutes

250g (9oz) unsalted organic butter

Before you begin, set a sterile glass storage container (see tip) to one side, then line a sieve with muslin (cheesecloth) and set this over a sterile glass jug.

Place the butter in a saucepan over a very low heat. The butter will begin to bubble and crackle, and a layer of white scum will slowly appear on the surface. Continue to heat the butter gently until it has liquefied completely and the bubbling and crackling have virtually ceased –this will take 10–15 minutes. The ghee should have a lovely buttery aroma and there should be no burning smell at any point.

Take the pan off the heat and gently pour the ghee through the lined sieve into the jug.

The jug should contain only the golden liquid and no white particles, which remain caught in the muslin. Discard the white solids. Transfer the ghee immediately to the storage container and allow to cool completely, then secure the jar with the lid.

The ghee will keep for several months. Store it in a cupboard or larder – it does not require refrigeration.

Tips

- To sterilize glass and stainless steel jars and ovenproof equipment, heat your oven to 140°C/120°C fan (275°F), Gas Mark 1. Clean the items to be sterilized (for this recipe, I upcycle jam jars) with plenty of hot, soapy water, rinse them in hot water, then put them, without drying, straight into the oven. Heat for 20 minutes to sterilize. Remove from the oven and allow to cool slightly before using.

- Always use clean utensils when using ghee, to prevent contamination of your stock and mould developing in your storage container.

Spiced pumpkin jam

This jam is known in Ayurveda as *kusmanda avaleha*. It is fabulous throughout autumn and winter after a long, hot summer. The taste of it is somewhere between a jam and a chutney. It helps to keep mucus clear from the body and dryness at bay, and also helps the body to retain a feeling of being grounded as you move into the shorter, cooler days. Use this jam on pancakes or stirred into porridge.

Makes 2 × 400g (14oz) jars
Preparation time 25 minutes
Cooking time 40–45 minutes

1.2kg (2lb 11oz) pumpkin, peeled, deseeded and chopped into small chunks
400ml (14fl oz) water
1.2kg (2lb 11oz) unrefined cane sugar
100g (3½oz) ghee (see page 196)
35g (1¼oz) ground ginger
25g (1oz) ground cumin seeds
10g (¼oz) ground cinnamon
10g (¼oz) ground black pepper
5g (¹⁄₈oz) ground coriander seeds
5g (¹⁄₈oz) ground cardamom seeds
50g (1¾oz) local honey

Put the pumpkin into a large saucepan with the measured water and bring to a boil, then reduce the heat to medium and simmer for approximately 25 minutes, until the water has reduced by half. Drain the cooked pumpkin through a sieve, retaining 1.2 litres (2 pints) of the water. Tip the pumpkin out of the sieve onto a tea towel and set aside to dry.

Meanwhile, pour the reserved pumpkin water into a saucepan with the sugar and bring the liquid to a boil. Cook over a high heat for 10–15 minutes, until the mixture begins to spit. Carefully dip a wooden spoon into the syrup, lift it out and watch the syrup drip back into the pan. If it seems thick and jam-like and flows in a stream, it is ready. If not, continue boiling for a further 2 minutes and test again.

While the pumpkin water is boiling, put the dried pumpkin into a mixing bowl and mash it with a potato masher (or whizz it using a food processor or blender) until smooth. Heat the ghee in a large frying pan over a medium heat, add the mashed pumpkin and fry gently for 5 minutes.

Once the pumpkin water mixture has the consistency of jam, mix in the fried pumpkin, boil for a further few minutes, until the jam has thickened a little more and when you perform the wrinkle test (see tip) it looks ready. Take the pan off the heat and mix in the spices. Allow the jam to cool so it reaches a temperature at which you can comfortably touch it, then add the honey. Mix until the consistency is uniform, then pour the jam into sterilized containers (see page 196 for sterilizing instructions). Store in a cool, dry place for up to six months.

Tips
- In order to check whether the jam is set, perform the wrinkle test. Put a plate in the refrigerator early on in the cooking process. When you think the jam is ready, drop some onto the cold plate, wait for it to be cool enough to handle, then push the edge of the jam with your finger. If it forms wrinkles, you know it is ready.

- This recipe is traditionally made with white gourd. Why not try growing some yourself?

Saffron pasta

Pasta is often made from durum wheat, which can be hard to digest for some people. But pasta can be made from most other flours. Its texture (based on the gluten content) and taste will vary as a result. Spelt flour is a good choice for those with a delicate digestion. Saffron is added here – it is warming and nourishing, which further promotes the nourishing quality of spelt wheat. The dish you make with this pasta will be ideal for those days that are physically demanding.

Serves 2
Preparation time 30 minutes, plus infusing
Cooking time 3–5 minutes

2 tablespoons water, plus extra as needed
tiny pinch of saffron strands
100g (3½oz) spelt flour (or use any flour of
    your choice), plus extra for dusting
1 teaspoon olive oil
pinch of unrefined salt

Put the measured water into a very small bowl and add a tiny pinch of saffron strands. Leave to infuse for 5–10 minutes.

Put the flour in a mixing bowl, add the oil and saffron water and strands and combine into a dough. You may need to add 2–4 tablespoons more water in order to encourage the flour to bind together – add 1–2 drops at a time so the dough does not become wet. Then knead and work the dough for around 10 minutes, until it is smooth and pliable. Engage all your senses in the process and enjoy the moments spent mindfully working the dough.

Divide the dough ball into 6 equal portions. Set your pasta machine to its widest setting, then dust it with flour. Pass 1 portion of dough through the machine to roll it. Fold the lengthened dough in half and roll the dough again. Continue to fold the rolled dough in half and roll it again, sprinkling the dough with flour as you go to prevent sticking, until the dough becomes pliable and smooth.

Now adjust the pasta machine to a narrower setting and pass the dough through it again. Continue rolling and folding the dough in this way, adjusting the pasta machine to a narrower setting each time so that the pasta becomes longer and thinner in depth.

Cut the sheet of pasta you have made into your desired shapes. Repeat with the remaining portions of dough.

To cook the pasta, bring a saucepan of water to a boil, add a tiny pinch of salt to the water along with the pasta, and cook for 3–5 minutes, until al dente. Drain the pasta, mix it with your chosen sauce and serve immediately.

Tips

• Dried pasta is a favourite staple food in many homes. Making fresh pasta offers a less processed option. It is not difficult to make and children love being involved in the process, especially if using a pasta machine. Kids also get a real buzz out of eating pasta they made themselves! If you do not have a pasta machine, you can roll the pasta using a rolling pin. Roll out each dough ball continuously to make it thinner and larger, turning it round constantly and rolling it from the centre of the circle outwards with increasing amount of pressure. Keep rolling until you reach the desired thickness and size.

• You can cut the pasta into largeish sheets to layer into a lasagne.

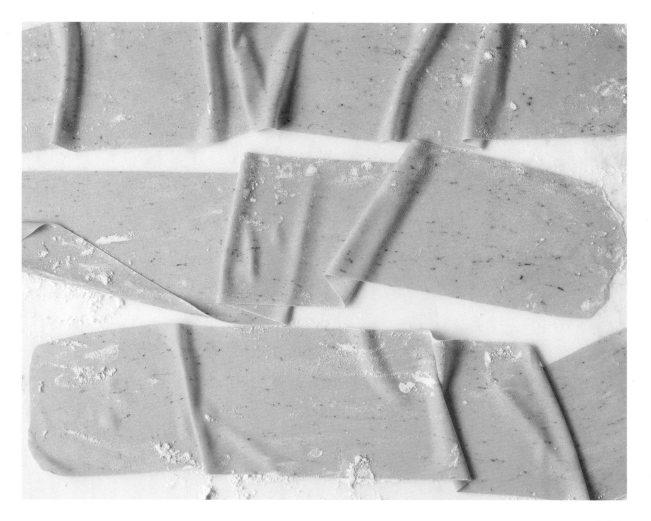

Sprouted chickpea hummus _____

This dish makes the fibre, protein and nutrient gems from chickpeas more bioavailable, and even increases the quantity of some of them. If chickpeas are sprouted prior to cooking, they lose more phytic acid during cooking than they would otherwise. (Phytic acid is an anti-nutrient that interferes with the body's absorption of minerals.) Sprouting and cooking processes also break down some of the complex sugars that the body's *agni* (digestive fire) finds difficult to process.

Serves 4
Preparation time 2–3 days
Cooking time 1 hour

To sprout
30g (1oz) dried chickpeas for sprouting
  (see pages 68–9)

For the hummus
75g (2¾oz) sprouted chickpeas
½ teaspoon garlic powder
2 tablespoons olive oil
1 teaspoon sesame seeds
few drops of lemon juice
small pinch of unrefined salt
up to 50ml (2fl oz) water
1 tablespoon chopped flat leaf parsley

Soak the dried chickpeas in water overnight in a sprouting jar. In the morning, drain the water, refresh the chickpeas with clean water and drain, then tip the top of the sprouting jar downward and rest it inside a bowl at an angle, so that any residual water will drain away. Place the bowl somewhere out of direct sunlight and leave to sprout. Over the next 2 days, refresh the sprouts with clean water twice a day. Sprouted tails should appear on the chickpeas by the end of this time.

Steam the sprouted chickpeas in a steamer pan for 45–60 minutes, until soft.

Allow the chickpeas to cool a little, then transfer to a blender jug. Add the remaining ingredients, except for the parsley, adding only 4 teaspoons of the measured water to begin with. Blitz the mixture until smooth, adding small amounts of water until you get the desired smooth consistency.

Transfer to a bowl and stir in the chopped flat leaf parsley.

Tips
• This hummus makes a great accompaniment to many dishes, and is perfect in wraps, on oat cakes or used as a dip. It can also be made with unsprouted chickpeas. Use 40g (1½oz) dried chickpeas, 75g (2¾oz) soaked and cooked weight, and double the cooking time. Alternatively, use 75g (2¾oz) canned chickpeas, adding the drained and rinsed canned beans directly into the blender jug.

• If you are not planning on serving it immediately, allow the hummus to cool completely, then store it in an airtight container and refrigerate. Use within 1 day.

Cumin labneh

A combination of cumin and healthy bacteria strains in yogurt makes this cheese wonderful for the digestive system. The live bacteria cultures ensure it is easy on the digestion. The cumin is a wonderfully savoury addition, but it can be omitted if you want to enjoy a plainer-tasting soft cheese, or replaced with any fresh seasonal herb, such as flat leaf parsley or coriander leaves. Its versatility means you can flavour it to accompany many different meals. The plain labneh can also be combined with sweet flavours, such as cardamom, cinnamon and honey, for a tasty treat.

Makes 3–4 portions
Preparation time Approximately 12 hours

200g (7oz) organic full-fat Greek yogurt
1 teaspoon lightly crushed cumin seeds

Combine the yogurt and cumin seeds in a bowl, then spoon the mixture into the centre of a square of muslin (cheesecloth). Gather the edges of the muslin together so that the yogurt forms a ball within it, then tie the neck of the ball with kitchen string, leaving a long tail of string.

Hang the ball, using the string, from a high cupboard door handle or something similar, so that the ball is suspended approximately 8cm (3¼in) above the countertop. Set a bowl underneath the yogurt ball to catch the whey that drops out of it. Leave to drip for 12 hours. I like to do this overnight so the cheese is ready to eat the next day.

After the 12 hours, release the labneh from the muslin. Store in an airtight container for up to 2 days.

Tips
- The leftover whey that drips into the bowl can be used in recipes in place of buttermilk or as part of the liquids in baking recipes. Add it to the Soda Bread (see page 110) in place of some of the water.

- Try making this cheese with keffir yogurt, to add even more gut-boosting bacteria.

201

For consultations or workshops/ Amnanda training with Anne Heigham
www.eatandbreathe.com
Instagram.com/anneheigham

To find a practitioner
In the UK
The APA
www.apa.uk.com

In the USA
National Ayurvedic Medical Association
www.ayurvedanama.org

For further ayurvedic educational learning
In the UK
The College of Ayurveda and Yoga Therapy
www.ayurvedacollege.org

In the UK and Europe
Amnanda
www.amnanda.eu

In the USA
The Ayurvedic Institute
www.ayurveda.com

For ayurvedic herb sourcing
In the UK
Essential Ayurveda
www.essentialayurveda.co.uk

Triveda
www.triveda.co.uk

Maharishi Ayurveda
www.maharishi.co.uk

In the USA
Banyan Botanicals
www.banyanbotanicals.com

vpk by Maharishi Ayurveda
www.mapi.com

Dr John Douillard's Life Spa Store
store.lifespa.com

Book resources
Textbook of Ayurveda (Volume 1): Fundamental Principles by Vasant Lad (Ayurvedic Press, 2002)

Textbook of Ayurveda (Volume 2): A Complete Guide to Clinical Assessment by Vasant Lad (Ayurvedic Press, 2007)

Textbook of Ayurveda (Volume 3): General Principles of Management and Treatment by Vasant Lad (Ayurvedic Press, 2012)

The Yoga of Herbs: An Ayurvedic Guide to Herbal Medicine by Dr David Frawley & Dr Vasant Lad (Lotus Press, revised edition 2001)

Encyclopedia of Herbal Medicine: 550 Herbs and Remedies for Common Ailments by Andrew Chevallier (Dorling Kindersley, 2016)

Music
Experience Yoga Nidra by Swami Janakananda

Om Mani Padme Hum by Sacred Earth

Deep Theta 2.0 (pt 13) by Steven Halpern

UK terms and their US equivalents _____

UK term	US equivalent
aubergine	eggplant
autumn	fall
bacon rasher	bacon strip
baking paper	parchment paper
baking sheet	cookie sheet
baking tray	baking sheet
bicarbonate of soda	baking soda
beetroot	beet
black-eyed beans	black eyed peas
casserole	casserole dish
cornflour	cornstarch
courgette	zucchini
full-fat milk	whole milk
green pepper	green bell pepper
infuse	steep
larder	pantry
loaf tin	loaf pan
pizza base	pizza crust
red pepper	red bell pepper
rocket	arugula
spring greens	collard greens
spring onions	scallions

Endnotes

Science of life

1 Haniadka R, Saldanha E, Sunita V, Palatty PL, Fayad R, Baliga MS. A review of the gastro-protective effects of ginger (Zingiber officinale Roscoe). *Food Funct.* 2013;4(6): 845–855. doi:10.1039/c3fo30337c

2 Arablou T, Aryaeian N, Valizadeh M, Sharifi F, Hosseini A, Djalali M. The effect of ginger consumption on glycemic status, lipid profile and some inflammatory markers in patients with Type 2 diabetes mellitus. *Int J Food Sci Nutr.* 2014;65(4):515–520. doi:10.3109/096374 86.2014.880671a

3 Mozaffari-Khosravi H, Talaei B, Jalali BA, Najarzadeh A, Mozayan MR. The effect of ground ginger supplementation on insulin resistance and glycemic indices in patients with Type 2 diabetes: a randomized, double-blind, placebo-controlled trial. *Complement Ther Med.* 2014;22(1):9–16. doi:10.1016/j.ctim.2013.12.017

Simple kitchen remedies

4 Zbuchea A. Up-to-date use of honey for burns treatment. *Annals of Burns and Fire Disasters.* 2014;27(1): 22–30.

Drinks

5 Lopresti AL, Drummond PD. Saffron (*Crocus sativus*) for depression: a systematic review of clinical studies and examination of underlying antidepressant mechanisms of action. *Human Psychopharmacology.* 2014. 29(6):517–27. doi: 10.1002/hup.2434

Staples and condiments

6 Plengvidhya V, Breidt F, Lu Z, Fleming HP. DNA Fingerprinting of Lactic Acid Bacteria in Sauerkraut Fermentations. *Applied and Environmental Microbiology.* 2007. 73(23): 7697–7702. doi: 10.1128/AEM.01342-07

Index _____

Acknowledgements

Firstly, I would like to thank my wonderful husband and
daughters for their tireless love and support. Our children,
especially, have been my best teachers. They have tasted,
read and inspired so much of this book.

I am also grateful to my wider family: my mother, who taught
me how to cook and introduced me to meditation, healing
and many other things from a young age; my late father, who
taught me that 'you create your own luck' and that anything
is possible with enough hard work, self-belief and timing; my
brothers, especially John who spent long hours in my kitchen
testing the recipes; and my 'in-law, second family', for all
their love, support and kitchen testing.

Without my beautiful clients this book would never have been
brought to life. At their request I began writing recipes in
2007 and they have received varying amounts of the content of
this book since that time.

I would like to thank all the brilliant teachers who have
gifted me the love and knowledge of Ayurveda over the years:
Dr Athique, Dr Palitha Serasinghe, Dr Marda, Dr Lad, Baba
Ramdas Swami, André Pammé and friend/teacher Andy Shakeshaft.

My gratitude also goes to Jane Graham-Maw, my agent, who
is so wise and brilliant; and to Kate Adams, who so deftly
sculpted this book into a much greater piece of work than
I ever had envisaged. Thanks also to Salima Hirani, for her
incredible copy-editing work, and to Leanne Bryan and Yasia
Williams-Leedham, for their creative talent in transforming
the manuscript into a visual delight.

Lastly, there are many friends without whose support and
encouragement along the way this book would not be here,
notably Laura and Tim James. Thank you all.